4x (9/10) 4/11

1x (6/08) 7/08

POWER-*of*-10

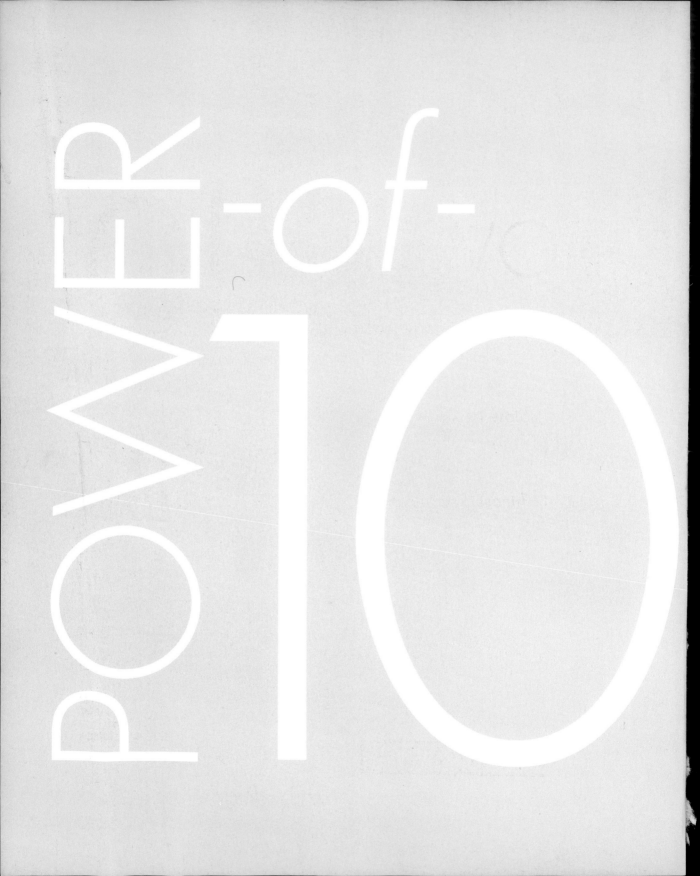

POWER-of-10

The Once-a-Week

Slow Motion

Fitness Revolution

Adam Zickerman

and Bill Schley

HarperResource

An Imprint of HarperCollinsPublishers

POWER-*OF*-10. Copyright © 2003 by Adam Zickerman and Bill Schley. All rights reserved. Printed in the United States of America. No part of this book may be used or reproduced in any manner whatsoever without written permission except in the case of brief quotations embodied in critical articles and reviews. For information, address HarperCollins Publishers Inc., 10 East 53rd Street, New York, NY 10022.

POWER-*OF*-10 is a trademark of Adam Zickerman and Bill Schley.

HarperCollins books may be purchased for educational, business, or sales promotional use. For information, please write: Special Markets Department, HarperCollins Publishers Inc., 10 East 53rd Street, New York, NY 10022.

FIRST EDITION

Designed by Richard Oriolo

Photographs by Ray Ellis

Photographs page 57 top courtesy © Strauss/Curtis/CORBIS
page 57 bottom courtesy © Bananastock/Wonderfile

Illustrations by Alexis Seabrook

LIBRARY OF CONGRESS CATALOGING-IN-PUBLICATION DATA HAS BEEN APPLIED FOR.

ISBN: 0-06-000888-1

03 04 05 06 07 WBC/QW 10 9 8 7 6 5 4 3 2 1

For my parents for being my deepest

and most enduring support

CONTENTS

PART I 10 SECONDS, 3 PILLARS, AND 1 WORKOUT TO CHANGE YOUR LIFE

PART II   THE POWER-*of*-10 STEP-BY-STEP WORKOUT

It gives me great pleasure to thank the many people who have made this book possible. At the top of the list are my dedicated and hardworking clients. They've become my friends and my greatest source of inspiration. I would like to give special thanks to my first client, Chuck Hordiner. The only thing greater than his faith in me is his big heart.

ACKNOWLEDGMENTS

I am extremely fortunate to work with an extraordinarily gifted staff at InForm Fitness, my studios in New York and Long Island. Over the years I've had the privilege to collaborate with some of the best exercise minds in the industry. I would like to give special thanks to Greg Anderson, co-owner, Ideal Exercise, Seattle, Washington; Ryan Hall, co-owner, One-to-One Personal Training and Clinical Exercise, New Orleans, Louisiana; John Nall and Patrick Ziebell, owners, Evolution Exercise and Spine Centers, Pewaukee and Wauwatosa, Wisconsin; David Landau, owner, Advanced Exercise Center, Hollywood, Florida; Rick Sullivan, owner, Personal Training Advantage, Bellmore, New York. I am eternally grateful to my mentors, Robert Francis, owner, Francis Strength/Medical, New York, and Robert Serraino, owner, Engineered Exercise, Washington, D.C. The models used to demonstrate the exercises in Chapter 6 are all actual clients. They are Malena Belafonte, Ron Storch, Don DiPaolo, and Matthew Rottino, and I am grateful to them for their willingness to volunteer long hours and work on location. A very special thank-you goes to Melena Belafonte, a client and busy fashion model, who brought a sense of order and professionalism to the photo shoot and who essentially waived her usual fee in support of the project. Even my photographer, Ray Ellis, is a client. His patience, expertise, and good humor made a very tedious project a real pleasure.

In addition I would like to thank Alvin Batista, owner, Glen Cove Health and Fitness, Glen Cove, New York, and Mike Ross, owner, All-Star Fitness, New York, for donating their facilities for the photo shoots.

Everyone I've had the pleasure to meet at HarperCollins has been so positive, supportive, and accessible, that I kept forgetting that I was working with a large global publishing house. To Janet Dery, thanks for believing in me enough to bring the book idea to HarperCollins. To Diane Reverand, a true visionary, thanks for offering me the book contract. To Greg Chaput, my talented editor, thanks for appreciating my sense of humor, and to Megan Newman, the voice of wisdom, thank you for calming all of our nerves.

I would like to give special thanks to Michael Carlisle, my trusted agent, and to Mei Mei Fox who was so helpful in organizing my thought processes at the beginning. I'd also like to thank Tracy Stopler, M.S., R.D., and Lisa Jubilee, M.S., C.N., for their wonderful insights and editorial recommendations for Chapter 3: Nutrition—The 2nd Pillar.

It is important for me to acknowledge two unsung heroes who, if it weren't for their faith and promotional efforts when my business was just getting started, I'd never have been offered the opportunity to write this book. Darla Senick-Shine, out of the goodness of her heart, was responsible for much of my early publicity. My good friend Adrienne Scordato was responsible for my PR Grand Slam, which blasted InForm Fitness to the moon. I am forever indebted to both of you.

A heartfelt thank you to Tracy Ann Longo, who thought of my studio's name, InForm Fitness, and who continues to have a powerful influence on my life.

Finally, this book is the result of a wonderful collaboration with my extremely talented cowriter, Bill Schley. I am lucky to have found a writer with such a knack for knowing what needs to be said. This book is as much his as it is mine.

—ADAM ZICKERMAN

McDonald's, Jiffy Lube, 1-Hour Photos: Americans love it their way—instant, easy, and effort-free. Sure enough, we're offered a countless variety of fitness solutions that on the surface seem to fit these requirements: miracle diets of all kinds, weight-loss pills, electric stimulators that shrink fat, and instant "ab" machines. But can there really be a *legitimate* workout/health program that deliv-

FOREWORD
Is This Too Good to Be True?

—FULTON C. KORNACK, M.D.,
Clinical Faculty in Orthopedic Surgery,
Harvard Medical School

ers full results in just a few minutes' time; that is doable and sustainable for the majority of us who lead busy lives, but still want to be fit and healthy without giving up our day jobs to spend hours at the gym?

There is such a program and it's called Power-*of*-10: It combines the principles of careful, slow-speed resistance training with lots of rest and a commonsense, palatable way of eating. It has the flexibility to fit into our lives and allow the pursuit of other "fun" recreational activities, while enabling the overall fitness we all desire. When I was first asked to evaluate Power-*of*-10 from a medical and orthopedic standpoint, I was doubtful about what seemed to be far too simple a plan. As an orthopedic surgeon, I had reviewed numerous workout regimens over the years to help rehabilitate and maintain both full-time and recreational athletes after injuries. In addition, patients constantly ask for recommendations for exercise programs to maintain musculoskeletal health, so they can perform their day-to-day activities in a more comfortable and effective way. Most of the regimens I've seen are capable of increasing fitness, yet the majority are too complex, time consuming, or potentially injurious. That means few patients would stick with them over time. And nothing works if you stop doing it. So, I approached Power-*of*-10 with my usual degree of scientific skepticism. However, as I examined its precepts, and listened to the stories of scores of individuals who swore to their success—and finally began the workout myself—I became convinced that the Power-*of*-10 philosophy was not only sound clinically but remarkably effective. It could be implemented safely by patients of all ages and abilities based on its 10-second, slow-speed cadences, its focus on workout quality over quantity, and its good sense philosophy of rest and nutrition.

It is an accepted fact in the field of orthopedics that resistance training (free weights, Nautilus, Bowflex, etc.) serves as the "core" of any successful, healthy conditioning program. This is true for people of all ages, from adolescents to senior citizens. Enhanced strength through resistance training helps to stabilize and protect the body's joints. This not only prevents injury, but improves performance. It has the added benefit of reducing stress on arthritic joints in the older population, which results in reduced symptoms and increased function. And for overall health, the lean muscle it generates plays a vital role in metabolizing and "burning" excess body fat. But again, the problem with most resistance programs is that they are too labor and time intensive; and those who do have the discipline tend to overtrain, leading to a host of potential traumas. My practice is filled with patients who in the process of building themselves up, are actually tearing themselves down with various traumatic and overuse injuries. The Power-*of*-10 program avoids all these pitfalls by utilizing a safe, nontraumatic mechanism that maximizes muscle strengthening in a way that enhances flexibility and overall conditioning. It provides a perfect platform to enhance additional aerobic programs or recreational athletic pursuits.

Power-*of*-10 is more than a resistance program, though. It is a philosophy of health and well-being that takes into account the other critical areas of fitness: nutrition and recovery. Without proper nutrition and without the opportunity for the body to recover and build on its efforts, the likelihood of injury and burnout becomes high. The basic tenets of the Power-*of*-10 nutrition philosophy fit what I call the "Ben Franklin" test: all good things in moderation and, occasionally, a few things in excess! The history and track record of American diets is abysmal. Extreme diets don't work. In contrast, Power-*of*-10 provides nutrition guidelines that combine proven concepts into a manageable and effective experience that one can continue over the long haul. It's not dieting, it's just a healthier way of eating every day. I can live with this!

As a doctor and a scientist, I am not interested in becoming a passionate disciple of the latest fad, but a user and recommender of a philosophy of life that will help my patients and myself to achieve the conditioning and overall health goals we all want. Power-*of*-10 is a well-researched and well-formulated program to help you reach your conditioning and general health goals in a remarkably achievable format. Read this book, follow its simple recommendations and you too will build your health and fitness on exercise, rest, and nutrition, The 3 Pillars of Power-*of*-10.

If you picked up a copy of *Newsweek* on February 5, 2001, you would've seen an article with a remarkable fitness story: *"For 10 years Dr. Philip Alexander ran 60 miles a week. . . . Then, five years ago, he really got serious about physical fitness. The 56-year-old Texas internist now spends just 20 minutes a week exercising, and he rarely soaks his shirt. Using weight machines, he works through a half-dozen muscle groups, diligently exhausting each one. Then he gets on with his life . . . that's not the best part. Alexander has shed some 20 unwanted pounds since switching regimens. . . . Could fitness be this simple?"*

INTRODUCTION

Could fitness be this simple?

Well, about 7 years ago, I quit my job, borrowed a few thousand dollars, and went on a personal quest to find out. This book is the result—along with two fitness centers, articles in major magazines, appearances on network television, and best of all, new lives for literally thousands of people I've trained who never believed they could have the beautiful, energized bodies they dreamed of, but now have. And every one did it with the 20-minute, once-a-week fitness program we call Power-*of*-10.

Yes, fitness not only can be this simple, you'll soon find it *needs* to be this simple to achieve the most dramatic results in the shortest time with the least risk of pain and long-term injury. Twenty years of research preceded this breakthrough in fitness training. Thousands of success stories now prove it. You'll meet them in this book. Give me 20 minutes, as little as once a week. Stick to the simple principles of Power-*of*-10, and you can have the other

10,058 minutes each week to relax and enjoy your hard, fit body with all its "perks" for the rest of your life.

COULD THIS BE YOU?

Believe me, all the folks who use Power-*of*-10, even the celebrities, are ordinary people. Time starved, stressed out, promising themselves every month they're going to get fit for a hundred reasons, but always procrastinating because, let's face it, it's just too hard. Everywhere you look, the conventional—I call it "pre-Power-*of*-10"—fitness industry says you've got to commit five or six days to weights and treadmills and aerobics each week, plus complicated, low-fat dieting, to have any success. I'd quit those programs because of the disgusting salad dressing alone! No question—these programs can work if you stick with them. But the reality is, for most of us, they're just impossible to keep up. The drop-out rate is over 85 percent! Not because we're lazy. But because today the world's too darned hectic to work out all week, every week, for the rest of our lives.

OUR LITTLE SECRET

Here's the secret I found. Over the years, I realized that everyone possesses one key asset like I do, and I suspect you do too, unless you're hooked up to a heart-lung machine: *everyone* has 20 minutes to make themselves healthy, once a week, two-thirds of an *I Love Lucy* rerun. And I'll say without exaggeration—of the many breakthroughs associated with Power-*of*-10's advanced form of exercise that you'll find in this book, this aspect turns out to be the most important breakthrough of all:

POWER-*OF*-10 IS SO FAST, CONVENIENT, SATISFYING AND SAFE, YOU SIMPLY WON'T WANT TO QUIT. *IT'S QUIT-PROOF!*

As any Power-*of*-10 user will tell you—this fact alone makes Power-*of*-10 the revolution that it is. Because no fitness program, no matter how great, can possibly work if you DON'T DO IT. I know how many exercise programs I've quit in my life after 3 weeks. What about you? Just imagine where you'll be 3, 6, 12 months and years from now when you've got a world-class fitness program that you actually stick with? That you actually look forward to after 5 to 7 days off? You'll be in buff-land, that's where you'll be. And you'll never want to go back.

THE 1-2-3 OF POWER-*OF*-10

Power-*of*-10 is made up of three parts I call "The 3 Pillars," which together make it a program for total body health and fitness. Each pillar is critical enough to have its own section in the book. The 3 Pillars are:

1 *Exercise*

2 *Nutrition*

and the one I consider our secret weapon because it's hardly mentioned in other fitness programs, yet it's as crucial as Pillar 1 and Pillar 2

3 *Rest & Recovery*

Trying to build a healthy body using quality exercise and nutrition, without quality rest and recovery, is like building a house without a foundation. Believe it or not, it's during rest that all the positive changes happen. By its very nature and design, Power-*of*-10, more than any other regimen, "positions" your body to get the rest and recovery it needs.

Pillar 1: Power-*of*-10 Exercise

Power-*of*-10 is, first and foremost, training with weights. An incredibly efficient, safe method of training with weights. You should know that today, everyone from the world's top fitness researchers to the Surgeon General agrees that weight training should be the main focus of every serious fitness routine. That's right, folks, weight-bearing exercise—not "cardio" exercise or aerobics. It's the key to strength, flexibility and, yes, even exercise-induced weight loss because it's the only way to build lean muscle mass, the body's most effective metabolizer of fat. It also has superior cardiovascular benefits when practiced correctly. If you're worried about "bulking up," just know that every cover model or movie star you love who has a hard, sculpted body—male or female—does it with weight training. Even top athletes who traditionally abstained from weights, like golfers, swimmers, and baseball players, do it now. In the next chapter, I'll explain why eliminating aerobic exercise from your workouts, except for fun, will actually make you healthier. But for now—please take it at face value that weights are the way to go for young and old alike.

HOW POWER-*OF*-10 DIFFERS FROM WEIGHT TRAINING YOU'VE SEEN BEFORE

The most notable difference between Power-*of*-10 and regular weight training is how slowly we move the weights in each exercise. Most lifters throw their weights up and down with a jerking, high-force motion. In Power-*of*-10, we slow ourselves down to a deliberate 10-second cadence: 10 seconds up and 10 seconds down. We don't stop at the top or bottom, so our muscles sustain a constant, steady load for about 5 to 8 repetitions. And we try to maintain perfect form during each 10-second motion—hence the name "Power-*of*-10." Finally, we choose a weight that will leave us "spent" by our last repetition. Moving the weights in this fashion "fires" the muscle fibers so deeply and completely, you'll notice a profoundly different feeling from any other workout the very first time you try it.

Pillar 2: What Is Power-*of*-10 Nutrition?

You don't need me to tell you—exercise alone can't do the job. The Power-*of*-10 workout will supercharge your body to burn calories and trim fat faster than you've ever experienced—but you can't get fit without intelligent nutrition.

Now for the good news. Because I didn't think you'd want another difficult diet plan like the hundreds out there that people start and quit every day. So here again I go back to the "Quit-Proof" principle that says no plan works if you don't do it. Like Power-*of*-10 Exercise, my Power-*of*-10 Nutrition plan is the most reasonable, simple, quit-proof method I know of—simply because I've watched more people succeed with its principles than any other. Exercise and nutrition is my profession. Eating is my passion. And this is the way I eat every day.

DON'T LAUGH. I WANT YOU TO EAT LIKE AN ANIMAL

Animals don't read charts, they don't count calories, and they don't diet. They do eat whole foods, avoid sugar, and eat meals throughout the day so they're never hungry. Their bodies burn up all the calories as they go. They drink tons of water. And occasionally, if an animal eats a big piece of double death-by-chocolate decadence cake, its body hardly notices. I'll show you Power-*of*-10 Nutrition in full detail in Chapter 3.

Pillar 3: This May Be the Most Valuable One of All

Rest & Recovery is the one great pillar of fitness that most programs completely neglect—yet it's probably the biggest success secret of Power-*of*-10. With Power-*of*-10, we literally *rest our way to success*. During exercise our bodies get temporarily weaker, not stronger. It's during rest that we recover and make *all* our gains. This is a huge, unspoken problem with even the most popular weight-training and exercise programs. Whether you're at the gym lifting or on the treadmill treading 6 days per week, you can't possibly have time for the rest your body needs. It's as if you were trying to grow a delicate crystal in water, but every day you come by and shake the glass. The crystal never has a chance. In the same way, too *much* exercise can be just as bad for you as too little. You reinjure yourself over and over, and never let your system reset itself and recover. You get muscle tears and strains, joint problems, chronic fatigue, and weakening of the immune system, so you get sick more often. Instead of building your body, you may be tearing it down. It amazes me how many dedicated exercisers hit the wall in their fitness programs and then stay there, month after month, without knowing why. They train harder and harder, when all they need is a little more rest.

NOW YOUR REST IS BUILT-IN

Needless to say, Power-*of*-10 is brilliantly conceived to let you get the rest you need in between workouts—five to seven days if you want it. During that time the pressure's completely off. While your body is nurturing and building itself, take the time when others are slaving on a treadmill somewhere to go on a nice walk, or meditate, or do yoga, or lie in a bubble bath, or read a book, or play a recreational sport like golf or tennis, or do absolutely nothing. You'll be doing absolutely everything to get out of your body's way and let it do its job, as it invariably will, if you balance the right exercise stimulus with the right opportunity to recover. In Power-*of*-10, if you reach a progress plateau, you don't do more exercise, you do more rest! In Chapter 4, I'll go over recovery in more detail, and offer the best tips and suggestions I know for enhancing recovery during your time between workouts.

HOW TO USE THIS BOOK

The first half of the book covers everything you'd ever need to know about Power-*of*-10 Exercise, Nutrition, and Rest & Recovery. The chapters aren't long because one of the nicest things about Power-*of*-10 is, it's not complicated! In the second half of the book you'll find all the step-by-step "how-to's." I've laid out and illustrated every exercise you'll ever need, suggested sample workouts, included easy nutrition guides, and much more. Everything for a complete life of fitness is contained in the pages ahead.

GETTING PSYCHED UP

Do you need any more psyching up to try a program that guarantees the healthy, hard body you've always dreamed of, by exercising 20 minutes, as little as once a week? I didn't think so. Let's go!

Jen Infurchia age 29
FLIGHT ATTENDANT

Burning the Candle at Both Ends—Until She Found Power-of-10 . . .

I'd been working out for years and I was sick of it! I was in a rut, my body was staying the same no matter how many days I slaved at the fitness center. And when I became a flight attendant, it just got to be impossible. I needed to stay trim and fit, yet the job

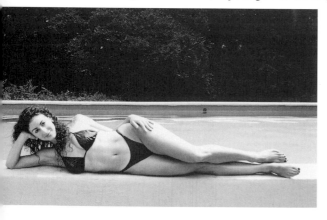

takes me to so many places on such short notice, keeping to a 4-day-a-week fitness routine is out of the question. I can get called on at 12 hours' notice and be gone for 10 days. I didn't know what to do anymore.

I tried Power-*of*-10 because a friend raved about it, and I was desperate to try anything. I have to admit now, I'm shocked that all the claims are true. I'd never felt such a depth of muscle work as I did the first workout. I loved the slow focus of the exercises right away. You just feel your muscles working. The after-workout feeling is tremendous, too. I'm totally spent, but exhilarated at the same time.

The difference between the controlled, smooth motion of Power-*of*-10 and the explosive lifting I was used to, made me instantly aware of how much safer the method was compared to normal training. Adam's right when he says you can be injury free, even with heavier weights.

When you try it for yourself, you'll see it makes total sense that you can do it just once a week because you fatigue such deep layers of muscle. You need the extra days to recover. I started feeling changes by my second workout. Just an energized feeling, like my muscles were soaking up the exercise. I started seeing new definition in the first few weeks.

Now that I've found Power-*of*-10, my scheduling problems are solved. I feel great because I'm getting the body I want without stressing about it. By the time my workout day comes around, I just can't wait.

POWER -of- 10

PART I

10 SECONDS, 3 PILLARS, AND 1 WORKOUT TO CHANGE YOUR LIFE

I've put this question to hundreds of people before they begin training: "What would you call an exercise technology, so advanced it . . .

■ builds lean muscle up to 50 percent faster than other exercise

■ supercharges your body to burn fat

STEP INTO THE EXERCISE FUTURE

■ cuts the chance of painful injuries to almost zero

■ builds cardio fitness without aerobic exercise

■ is so efficient, it requires as little as 20 minutes, once a week?"

I then proclaim, "You wouldn't call it exercise, you'd call it *FUTURE-CISE!*" And they say, "Future-cise? That is the *dumbest* name I've ever heard. . . . But, is the rest true?"

Yes, it is, or you wouldn't be reading this book, and thousands of people wouldn't be learning to train this way. When you apply modern science to any endeavor—from spaceships to sports activity—you discover breakthroughs in the technology of doing things. Take skiing. Picabo Street's not doing 65 mph on old wooden, long boards with bear-trap bindings. Her Kevlar composite parabolic skis and titanium bindings have revolutionized what she can do on skis. Now, remember when exercise was two fat guys in those old movies throwing a medicine ball at each other's gut? Exercise science has undergone the same evolution. Twenty years ago, researchers began experimenting with weight training, and the result is the core technology of Power-*of*-10.

WEIGHT TRAINING IS THE KEY TO THE KINGDOM

I want to start by thanking America's top fitness experts and the authors of today's best-selling workout books. They've written hundreds of pages and made millions of people aware of a major theme of *this* book—which means I only have to cover it in a page and a half. The theme is that, after thirty years of being told by the establishment that fitness is a matter of endless aerobics sessions on a squeaking treadmill, America is not fit, not lean, not in shape, and not losing weight. The truth, the experts agree, is that the key to fitness and weight loss is resistance training with weights. And after devoting my whole career to fitness and health, I'll second that emotion. Weights are the shining path. The reason's really quite simple. Only resistance training with weights builds lean muscle mass. By comparison, aerobics builds virtually none. Only lean muscle mass can change the shape of your body to the trim, curvaceous, or muscular form you want. For women who are afraid of bulking up, lean muscle actually makes their body profile smaller because muscle is more compact.

25 AEROBIC WORKOUTS PER MONTH, WHILE YOU SLEEP

But here's the best part: lean muscle mass requires the burning of energy—that is, it has to burn calories just to sustain itself in your body. So the more lean muscle you have versus fat, the more calories you burn while you sit, while you relax, and while you sleep. A lot more. Three extra pounds of lean muscle burns about 10,000 extra calories a month, just sitting around! Add it up. Since aerobic exercise like jogging burns only about 100 calories per mile, and a typical aerobic workout burns 100 calories every 15 minutes, having 3 extra pounds of muscle burns as many calories as running 25 miles per week, or doing 25 aerobic workouts per month without leaving your couch! It's really amazing. Your metabolism is revved up by lean muscle to do this all by itself. You become a fat-burning furnace. Scientists have also found that building lean muscle has superior cardiovascular benefits. By building muscle mass, the body has to grow new microvascular capillary networks to serve those muscles. This makes the heart increase its efficiency to service the expanded network. Since the heart is a muscle, increasing efficiency means getting stronger. And again, the heart exercises to service capillaries 24 hours a day not just when you're on a treadmill. Increasing fitness by weight training has also been shown to lower blood pressure, a good indicator that the heart becomes more efficient at delivering oxygen to your muscles as a direct result of weight-bearing exercise.

AEROBICS REALITY—WHAT THE FITNESS CHAINS WON'T TELL YOU

Nobody is saying you should quit aerobics altogether if it's something you like to do for fun or to relieve a little stress. I love basketball and bike riding. Just do it as a supplement to weight training, never as a substitute. Unlike weight training, which speeds your whole fat-burning metabolism, the moment you stop the treadmill, you stop burning the calories. Aerobics does little to change your body composition because it not only fails to burn much fat, build muscle mass, or boost your metabolism, it can even reduce muscle mass. And there's another side of the coin that experts are increasingly worried about. Repetitive stress injuries don't only come from pounding keyboards with your fingertips each day. What about pounding a road with the balls of your feet year after year, or putting hundreds of pounds of pressure on your knees with every pedal stroke, five thousand times a bike ride? Our joints and tendons were never designed for that. The fact is, physiologists are starting to warn that the current generation of compulsive cardio trainers may be setting themselves up for an epidemic of chronic joint and connective tissue injuries as they get older. A large percentage of regular joggers develop a serious joint or tissue injury over the course of 3 years. What's the point of keeping your muscles in shape while you're young, if you'll have to use a cane to get up the stairs in 10 years? The point is, we need exercise that wears out our muscles each workout—not our joints and connective tissues.

IF WEIGHT TRAINING IS SO GREAT, WHY POWER-*OF*-10?

Because Power-*of*-10 *is* weight training in a remarkably efficient, more concentrated form. It's been shown to be safer, to work faster to change your body composition, and, best of all, you can do the entire program just once a week in about 20 minutes if you want. Regular weight training is great if you know you have time for an hour in the gym, 4 to 6 days per week. But if achieving your goal once a week in less than half an hour appeals to you—keep reading. You'll find that Power-*of*-10 is so advanced, it's *Future-Cise*! Oops—I mean it's the *Future of Exercise*!

BIRTH OF A REVOLUTION—THE DISCOVERY OF THE
SLOW-MOTION PRINCIPLES BEHIND POWER-*OF*-10

The principles used in Power-*of*-10 came mostly from the work of two pioneers of resistance training in the 1970s and 80s—Arthur Jones, inventor of the famed Nautilus weight machines, and Ken Hutchins, who developed a method of training that he later trademarked as SuperSlow. Arthur Jones's Nautilus machines, the first designed to follow the body's natural movements, are the precursors to all the equipment you see in today's gyms. He is also known as the father of High Intensity Training, or HIT, which showed that brief, intense training in which you perform just one set until muscle failure, increases muscle mass far more quickly than long sessions of multiple sets.

In the early 1980s, Jones asked Ken Hutchins to run a clinical trial to see if his Nautilus machines could help women with osteoporosis regain lost bone density and lost mobility through developing increased muscle mass. Hutchins realized that regular Nautilus training was too dangerous. Its high-force, explosive HIT movements would risk breaking fragile bones. Understanding that force is a function of speed, Hutchins decided to drastically slow things down. He had his subjects move the weights almost in slow motion. What he discovered would lead to a revolution in the safety and effectiveness of modern weight training. Indeed, slow motion was safer—it eliminated injuries, as Hutchins intended, but he also found that the women gained muscle mass far more rapidly than with conventional weight training. When Hutchins tried slow motion on healthy people, he discovered the rest of the story. The protocol was more efficient because it actually took the high-intensity method to even more of an extreme without the dangers and difficulties of heavy weights at high force. Moving slowly worked a greater number of muscle fibers, eliminated wasted momentum, and allowed trainees to maintain proper form and complete control. The exercise was so efficient, there was no reason to do multiple sets. By working to full muscle fatigue in just one short set, people were getting all the benefits of a full workout, in a fraction of the time spent at the gym. In fact, you could build muscle mass dramatically with less than half an hour of training a week.

EXERCISE "FLIPS A SWITCH" IN EACH MUSCLE. WAIT'LL YOU SEE WHAT POWER-*OF*-10 DOES

Here's the best physiological explanation for why Power-*of*-10 is so incredibly efficient. As you know, if you've taken high school biology, fatiguing muscle during exercise causes temporary, microscopic injuries to muscle cells. As the muscle makes repairs, it reinforces itself for the next injury by adding additional, thicker fibers, thus making it stronger than before. In fact, exercise fatigue causes the release of a "growth factor" chemical that "flips a switch" in the DNA that lines

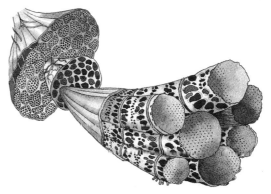

A muscle is a bundle of millions of fibers like these.

the muscle cell walls, causing the muscles to begin replicating themselves. New fibers attach to the injured cells, making them thicker and stronger so they can cope better with the next challenge. Again, one great benefit of this natural muscle repair process is that it takes huge amounts of stored energy to perform; hence we burn calories and fat.

POWER-*OF*-10 FLIPS ALL THE SWITCHES AT ONCE

Here's the difference with Power-*of*-10. Just like the common belief that we only use about 10 percent of our brains, conventional, high-speed weight training fires only a relatively small percentage of our muscle cells in each workout. Our goal *should* be a workout that can fatigue or "flip the switch" in 90 to 100 percent of our targeted muscle cells—the switch that makes them start rebuilding automatically. Once we've triggered all our muscle cells, it's time to go home from the gym. There are simply no more cells left to stimulate, and if we keep exercising, all we can do is keep reinjuring them. It's just that simple—when all the switches are flipped, we stop and let the cells do what they do best: build our bodies from within over the next 5 to 7 days. All they ask of us is to give them enough rest and nutrition and they'll perform miracles.

Now, what if you could stimulate all the muscles in one incredibly efficient workout? That's right. You'd be done in one workout! And that's exactly what Power-*of*-10 can do.

THE 10-SECOND SECRET

The key to Power-*of*-10 is the deliberately slow, controlled, 10 second upward and 10 second downward movement of the weights in each repetition, or "rep." Since each repetition is one up-down cycle, a complete rep takes 20 seconds, during which you focus intently on correct form. Moving at this speed eliminates any chance of cheating with the weight's momentum. One hundred percent of the work is done by your muscles. You spend about 90 to 120 straight seconds like this, firing deeper and deeper and deeper layers of muscle fibers until, suddenly, you're spent. Believe me, it's a different sensation from other workouts. You feel that you've thrown every switch you have. Your work will be over for that whole muscle group in one set. Five to six more sets *max* to cover your other major muscle groups and you're ready to go home. Your muscles are now in an internal body-building mode that will last for the next 5 to 7 days if you don't interfere.

Now compare what I've just described to the way you see most people throwing weights around in the gym and you'll be struck by the contrast. The average conventional set of 10 reps lasts just 15 to 20 seconds. Since the trainee is most concerned with completing a number of reps, he or she jerks the weight up and down as quickly as possible to get the set over with. Simple momentum from the moving weight does a great percentage of the work, stealing the benefits. And improper form causes the weight to be supported by joints and bones during key parts of the rep, rather than by muscles alone. It's kind of like lighting a fireplace log. Touch a flame to it and keep taking it away—it'll never catch. But hold the flame against it for 2 minutes straight and you'll start the self-sustaining chain reaction called fire.

WHY A POWER-*OF*-10 WORKOUT CAN BE SO SHORT— JUST 20 TO 25 MINUTES

Six exercise sets are simply all your body needs and, frankly, all it can take before you have fatigued all the muscles and switched them into rebuilding mode. If you accomplish six 120-second sets, it adds up to 12 minutes of pure exercise. The best way to do the workout is to go from set to set without stopping until you are finished. So, if you add another 10 minutes to get from one machine to the next, you come up with 20 minutes on average. And because the movements are so smooth and gradual, you never subject your muscles, joints or connective tissues to sudden, jolting forces. In fact, one of the reasons Power-*of*-10 is so much shorter than other workouts is that it requires no traditional 10- to 15-minute warm-up period. You simply start cold into the first exercise, and your body warms itself up immediately in the first 2 to 3 reps. The warm up is built-in—saving you time and saving you injury because you automatically get a proper warm-up every time—even when you're rushed at the gym.

THE BIG SAFETY BONUS

The combination of the built-in warm-up plus slow, smooth nonjerking movements provides a major fringe benefit that many Power-*of*-10 enthusiasts find as important as any other. Injuries somehow cease to exist when you do Power-*of*-10. Conventional weight lifting at conventional speeds subjects the joints, ligaments, and connective tissues—not to mention the muscles themselves—to hundreds of pounds of brutal force. No matter how careful I was when I used to train this way—even when I tried lighter weights—I was chronically injured. A pull here, a strained tendon or inflamed joint there. And it got worse as I got older. I hated having to stop working out, sometimes for months at a time and giving up all my hard earned gains because I had to let a right brachialis muscle heal or my shoulder joints were too painful to move. Injuries also happen when we don't rest enough between workouts and muscles weaken and reinjure themselves. Both the force problem and the rest problem are completely eliminated by Power-*of*-10. It's the only serious protocol I know that purposely wears out your muscles but never your joints, tendons, ligaments, or bones. You can't say that for four- to six-day weight-training programs, and you especially can't say it for aerobics.

NOW WE'RE ABOUT TO BEGIN

At this point, I'm hoping your mental door of acceptance is propped open—just enough for you to consider that the thousands of us who exercise with Power-*of*-10 principles are not hallucinating, that we really do get the benefits I'm talking about, and that we wouldn't work out any other way. Now I'll show exactly how to do Power-*of*-10 yourself—starting today if you want to. The next three chapters cover The 3 Pillars of total fitness: Power-*of*-10 Exercise, Power-*of*-10 Nutrition, and Power-*of*-10 Rest & Recovery. They'll show you the entire protocol that will change your fitness life—step by step, rep by rep. I hope you're getting excited.

David Sparrow age 38

MAGAZINE EDITOR AND WRITER

"It Seemed Too Good to Be True, Until I Tried It Myself . . ."

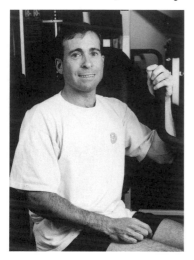

When I was assigned to do an article for *Men's Journal* magazine about a new type of weight training that promised to make me fitter and stronger in less than 30 minutes a week, I was skeptical. Put simply, it seemed too good to be true. I'd always been led to believe that the only way to accomplish this was to visit the gym and pump iron at least 3 times a week. I decided the best way to test the merits of the Power-*of*-10 was to try it out myself. Within a few sessions I was hooked, and a year later, I still am. Although I'd lifted weights before, they were always an afterthought to my cardio work. And the reason for that was simple: there was no structure to my lifting. My reps were lightning quick and I never seemed to make any progress either in adding weight to the stack or adding muscle mass to my runner's build.

The Power-*of*-10 was different from the start. I loved the whole vibe of the workout—how my taking deep, rhythmic breaths during exercises helped me maintain control, how I could close my eyes and achieve a Zen-like focus, how knowing that it would be over within half an hour gave me inspiration to get through the task at hand. There are no breaks between exercises, and I'm usually exhausted when it's done. Since I began working with Adam, I've more than doubled the weight I lift on every machine. I'm now leg-pressing 560 pounds, which is four times my body weight! Within 2 months of beginning the Power-*of*-10, my wife, Darcy, noticed that my stomach muscles were starting to form a six-pack. And over time, she's said that my body fat has virtually disappeared. Friends have noticed my better definition, too. So have I. While I'll never be a he-man, my legs and arms are stronger and look bigger. I no longer bother with the stationary bike—it's not necessary when doing the Power-of-10. My most recent checkup proved as much: my cholesterol is down 10 percent to 132, and my blood pressure dropped from 122/80 to 102/74.

Nothing else in my diet, lifestyle, or exercise regimen has changed to explain these results. It's all due to the Power-*of*-10. That's why I'm truly glad I gave the program a try. So should you.

And now, through the legal authority vested in me as your author, I pronounce you ready to begin your new fitness life. If you relax and enjoy the trip, I guarantee you'll succeed because there's not a single thing in the next few pages that you can't do.

EXERCISE— THE 1ST PILLAR

POWER-*OF*-10 "QUICK-START"

Here's the 1-minute perspective on everything you need to know. Then we'll cover the few details that make the protocol truly effective. But before you go on, let me say this: some folks apparently feel that people who do Power-*of*-10 get so into it, it's like a religion. That's ridiculous. I don't know where they get that idea.

The 10 Commandments of Power-*of*-10

1 **THE SPEED COMMANDMENT**—Thou Shalt Perform Repetitions That Are 10 Seconds Up, 10 Seconds Down.

2 **THE BREATHING COMMANDMENT**—Thou Shalt Not Hold Your Breath, but Shall Breathe Freely and Evenly, Always.

3 **THE MOTION COMMANDMENT**—Thou Shalt Never Jerk the Weights Up or Down, but Shall Be Smooth and Constant.

4 **THE NUMBER OF REPS COMMANDMENT**—Thou Shalt Do the Number of Reps It Takes for Your Muscles to Run Out of Gas, Until You Cannot Do Another One; Then Try to Push for 10 More Seconds.

5 **THE NUMBER OF EXERCISES PER WORKOUT COMMANDMENT**—Thou Shalt Be Done After About 6 Different Exercises or Sets If You Work Out Correctly.

6 **THE CORRECT WEIGHT COMMANDMENT**—Thou Shalt Choose a Weight Where You Reach Your Limit at About 6 to 8 Reps When You First Begin Training.

7 **THE NO-STOPPING COMMANDMENT**—Thou Shalt Move Quickly from Exercise to Exercise Until the Workout Is Done.

8 **THE FOCUS COMMANDMENT**—Thou Shalt Have a "Zen-like" Focus at All Times to Concentrate on Form, Motion, and Speed.

9 **THE NUMBER-OF-WORKOUTS-PER-WEEK COMMANDMENT**—Thou Shalt Do About One Workout Per Week—Resting in Between for 5 to 7 days; However, You Mayest Do a Lighter Workout, Twice a Week, If You Feel Like It.

10 **THE EQUIPMENT COMMANDMENT**—Thou Shalt Do Best and Be Safest If You Use Machines; However, I'll Also Show You How to Do It at Home.

You could take these 10 Commandments, go right to the gym, and instantly do yourself more good with less risk than any conventional weight-training workout. But believe me, the specific pointers that follow will guarantee your success to a much higher level. Read on for the simple tips and refinements, made over two decades, that are the keys to all that Power-*of*-10 has to offer.

SECRETS AND TECHNIQUES THAT MAKE ALL THE DIFFERENCE

1. The Right Speed and Motion

Again, the core of the Power-*of*-10 protocol is the 10-second motion each time we move the weight—10 seconds up and 10 seconds down—making a full repetition, or rep, last 20 seconds. Once we begin a set of reps, we never stop to rest, even for a second, at the top or the bottom. Instead, just before our limbs reach what we call "lockout" at the top of a motion, we seamlessly reverse ourselves and begin back down. Likewise, at the bottom, just before "bottoming out," we smoothly, seamlessly begin pushing the weight back up. Every rep is like a continuous circle—I call it the "circle of power"—that continues at the same, smooth, constant speed until the end of the set.

The Circle of Power

This continuously smooth, up-and-down technique is so important, it's worth practicing with almost no weight at first until it becomes second nature. Position yourself in a weight machine and from the starting point, begin moving the weight stack in the positive or "lifting" direction. The start of motion is CRUCIAL. Practice pushing so gradually that the movement of the weight stack is almost imperceptible. The goal is to eliminate all momentum so your muscles do 100 percent of the work. We absolutely never jerk or "blast" the weight into motion as in regular weight training—and thus we eliminate the high-speed forces that cause most weight-training injuries. Instead, I want you to sque-e-e-eze the weight into motion and begin to count the 10 seconds to yourself. You should be at the halfway point as you hit number 5. Just before you get to the top of the motion and full arm extension—or lockout—start back in the negative direction. Avoid locking out because it puts extra pressure on your bones and joints, and we don't want the weight resting on your

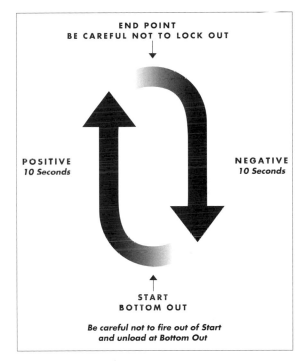

Circle of Power

bones, we want it held by muscle for the entire set. Power-*of*-10 at its best is "filet of exercise"—it works out pure, concentrated muscle cells, never wears out joints, ligaments, or other connective tissue. So again, when you reverse your motion, make a smooth U-turn at the top of the circle. Then count your way smoothly back down to the bottom of the motion where you started the rep. Make the same U-turn at the bottom and start back up without resting or "unloading" your muscles. Continue this way until the end of the set. That's the basic circle of power you'll use from now on.

2. Completing the Perfect Rep

In Power-*of*-10, you do such a small number of reps in each workout, it stands to reason that every rep counts. When you're really advanced, you'll get so efficient, you can actually do less and less reps and still get the same benefits. Some of the most rippling Power-*of*-10 people I know do as little as 15 total reps per workout, once a week! At 20 seconds per rep, that's a grand total of 5 minutes of actual exercise, folks, no kidding. But boy, those are some perfect reps. So what we're after is quality—that is, perfect form and deep muscle fatigue—not quantity. It's the little things that make the big difference.

First and Foremost, Breathe

In business you always hear location, location, location. In Power-*of*-10 it's breathe, breathe, breathe! Never hold your breath. I know many of you are thinking, "What—he has to tell me to breathe? Last time I noticed, I think I was breathing." Yes, but there's a big difference between the shallow, unconscious, irregular breaths most people take and the big, deep, full breaths that will superoxygenate your hardworking muscles and produce the most efficient workout. Yoga has promoted this concept for thousands of years. These breaths are called "belly" breaths. Unless you're conscious of your breathing, you'll have the tendency to hold your breath. And that's probably Power-*of*-10's biggest no-no. It can raise your blood pressure and strain other organs, particularly the heart. Careful breathing keeps your blood pressure down. It keeps you more relaxed and focused. It helps you keep a smoother, more regular cadence. And it sends more vital oxygen to your muscles so they take the maximum time to fail, thus fatiguing the most cells. All I want you to do is remember to breathe freely, deeply, in and out, during every rep. Proper breathing is the cornerstone of your success.

Get Into a Zen-Like Focus

The more you concentrate on your target muscles and relax the rest of your body, the more perfectly efficient your reps will be. At the gym, you'll see all the civilians grimacing and grunting and squirming their way through the hardest reps. Now that you're on the Power-*of*-10 team, you're above such amateur behavior. A grimacing face never lifted a pound of weight. Keep your face relaxed, your breathing steady, your speed constant, and hold to proper form. Focus on those target muscles. It's only a few seconds so make them count.

And Last, but Most Important of All . . .
I want you to fail. This concept deserves its own section, so here it is.

3. At the End of Each Set, You Must Reach "Muscle Failure"

I know it sounds like reverse logic but in Power-*of*-10, you succeed mostly by "failing." In other words, on the last rep of each set, you shouldn't be able to move the weight anymore. You should be spent. When you think about it, it makes perfect sense. The only way you know you've fatigued every muscle cell—that you've flipped 90 to 100 percent of those DNA switches that start the magical muscle rebuilding process so you can take the rest of the week off—is to go to your exercise limit, or "muscle failure." You're there when you've fired all your muscle cells and you don't have any more to lift with. While all your reps are important—the last rep in the set, the failure rep, pushes the benefits off the charts. So in Power-*of*-10, muscle failure is the thing we strive for and practice and get better and better at achieving with time. In the beginning, I just want you to get up to the failure threshold and see what it feels like. Later you can push as far as you want into this zone of body transformation, knowing that every extra second you spend over the threshold, still pushing against the immovable weight without quitting, gives you enormous added benefits. It's like a fireworks grand finale—millions of extra cells start igniting all at once, producing a crescendo of results.

The Simple Way to Fail

In a minute, I'll show you how to pick the right weight to start with and how many reps you're going to do in each set. But for now, let's say you're using a weight where you run out of steam on the sixth rep. That means, you start the sixth rep and you just can't finish. The weight stays where it is and stops moving. In conventional training, you'd drop the weight on the floor. But in Power-*of*-10, this is the potato skin where all the vitamins and minerals are. We don't waste it. When the weight refuses to move any further, *we simply keep pushing for 10 extra seconds.* Call it the "Threshold Push." During those few seconds the weight may not be moving; but no matter, it's your trying that counts. The more the better. At the end of the Threshold Push, we let the weight down slowly at our normal, controlled speed.

Now please note, a 10-second Threshold Push is our rule of thumb. But it's not set in stone. In the beginning, just get to the threshold and keep pushing for a second or two to see what it's like. With practice, you'll quickly find yourself pushing longer and longer, for 10 seconds or more, depending entirely on how you feel and how much intensity you want in your workouts.

What Muscle Failure Feels Like

As your muscles reach failure, you'll begin to feel a normal sensation that I call "burn." The burn goes from a slight discomfort to fairly uncomfortable, to *really* uncomfortable the longer you continue, so your natural tendency is to want to stop. But believe me, as you practice reaching failure, this feeling becomes like an acquired taste. You not only get more and more used to it, you actually find yourself not feeling physically and psychologically satisfied until you've pushed yourself to the limit and experienced a "really good burn." For one thing, you'll know you've given yourself a 100 percent effective workout. And for another, the post-workout feeling when you've reached muscle failure and flipped all your switches is different. It's awesome. It's a relaxed, whole body "glow" that really has to be experienced.

Fear of Failure? Fuggedaboudit!

If Power-*of*-10 wasn't within everyone's ability, it wouldn't be one of the fastest growing exercise methods in America. If my own mother can do it, anyone can. But if you're concerned about pushing your limits, because maybe you haven't done that before, here's what to keep in mind when it comes to failure induced burn:

1   The burn is entirely voluntary. *You* decide how many seconds you want to continue your Threshold Push, the place where the burn is, depending on how intense and efficient you want your workout to be. In the beginning, go easy.

2   The burn stops the instant you stop.

3   The burn period is incredibly good for you. One reason we normally recoil from pain or discomfort is that we instinctively feel it signals danger or impending harm to our

bodies. But with Power-*of*-10, it's the by-product of doing something tremendously healthy for our bodies. Remember, during the last failure rep when we feel the burn, the weight is essentially stationary. Injuries don't happen when weights are stationary. Injuries happen when weights are moving quickly with great force. Compared to Power-*of*-10's rate of injury, running on a treadmill is dangerous.

As people practice Power-*of*-10, they adapt to the feeling they get during the Threshold Push—generally deriving deeper and deeper satisfaction the more they advance past the threshold. Everyone finds the threshold that works for them. You will, too.

4. Doing Your First Workout

Picking the Exercises
Over 35 of the best exercises, along with suggested workouts, are shown step-by-step in Part II of this book.

Power-*of*-10 is a whole body workout, so you'll do both upper and lower body; back and front each time. You'll use both "compound exercises" to work multiple muscle groups, and "simple exercises" that isolate one or two muscles at a time. Again, you'll only be doing 5 or 6 exercises total in the whole workout, so you need to cover the full body. In Part II, I've illustrated all the different exercises you'll ever need, plus suggested workout combinations for all levels.

Picking the Right Weight and Number of Reps
Once you've had practice and are gaining strength, an optimum set will be just 4 to 6 reps. But in the beginning—even if you're already in shape—I want you to pick a lighter weight where you fail by about the eighth rep. Since each full rep lasts 20 seconds, that means you'll fail in about 160 seconds. It takes 3 to 4 workouts of trial and error on the different machines before you settle on the perfect weight. But I promise, after a few workouts, *the right weight will find you*! During this ramp-up period, you're practicing your circle of power, remembering your breathing, getting comfortable with the speed, and learning what it feels like to reach failure. The first time, pick any reasonable looking weight and start your set. You may blow right past 8 reps to 10 or more. Or you might konk out at 5. Next workout, add a few pounds if the weight is too light, or

remove a few if it's too heavy; it's as simple as that. Within a few workouts, you'll zero in on that weight that allows you 8 reps before failure. From there, we start measuring regular progress.

Stick with the 8-rep count for a while until you're really feeling comfortable and confident with the program. When you get stronger and more experienced, 6, 5, 4, or even 3 reps may be preferable in terms of time and effectiveness. What matters most is that you keep good form, consistent speed—and that you take yourself to muscle failure.

Measuring Your Progress

In any kind of training, you must have a way to measure progress, not only to see if you're getting stronger, or just maintaining a desired level of fitness, but to gauge whether there are problems with your program that need adjustment. For example, sometimes it's possible to feel a loss of stamina or energy over a number of workouts. You'd know that because you'd suddenly be failing in a shorter time, after fewer reps. In that case, it's time to make an adjustment. Most commonly, I'd prescribe another day or two of rest between workouts, because negative gains generally mean you're overtraining and need more recovery time. But hitting a plateau or reaching failure sooner than usual can also mean you're not eating properly, or not sleeping well, or that you're stressed out at work. You need to keep all the "healthy" variables as consistent as possible to make the most accurate adjustments and to best analyze your progress.

Counting Time Until Failure

In conventional weight training, people count sets and reps. A typical goal might be "3 sets of 10." Get to your number, and quit. Power-*of*-10 is completely different. Our goal is to get to muscle failure, regardless of the rep count, and then keep pushing past the threshold for a few seconds. The way we measure progress is simple: we measure what we call Time Until Failure, or TUF; that is, how many seconds we can move a certain weight until we fail or run out of gas. There are two ways to time yourself—either with a stopwatch like those found on any digital wristwatch or by counting to yourself. Those who prefer a stopwatch like it because they don't have to think about counting during the set and they never forget the number. You just hit the button on the watch and start the first rep. Reach failure and hit the button again. If your goal is to fail at 6 reps and the watch says 120 seconds, you're right on with that weight. If your time increases in the next workout, you know you're taking longer to fail and you're getting stronger. Now, if you like to keep to a 6-rep Time Until Failure, just add a little more weight. You're making progress.

Other people like to count to themselves without a watch. The simple way to do that is to keep a mental count of each rep as you go through the set. Since every full rep is a uniform 20 seconds, all you're doing by keeping count is tracking the number of 20-second increments until your muscles fail. If your goal is a 6-rep TUF, and you complete 6, great. If in the following weeks you hit 8 or 9 before failure, you're getting stronger and can add more weight, bringing your count back down again to a 6-rep TUF. Counting to yourself is not as exact as using the watch, but it works fine for measuring progress. Do it either way.

The Right Number of Exercises

Six exercises is the average number for once-a-week workouts, although, depending on your personal preference, your intensity level, and your experience, you can do as few as 4 exercises or as many as 8. Generally, if you take yourself to failure, your body will tell you it's ready to rest after 6 exercises. You might pick 3 upper body exercises and 3 lower; or 4 and 2—it's up to you. All this is covered in Part II. As the Seventh Commandment states, the very best way to go through your routine is to do exercise after exercise without stopping until the entire workout is completed. This raises the overall intensity level and produces deeper muscle fatigue. It also enables the workout to be as short as it is. Six 120-second exercises adds up to 12 minutes of pure exercise. A minute or so to get from machine to machine adds another 5 to 8 minutes, giving you a 20-minute workout. Once again, as you get really advanced and are willing to crank up the intensity, shorter and shorter workouts can still get you to failure. As I said earlier, it's not uncommon for experts to maintain incredible fitness with a routine of five 3-rep exercises, once a week. That's *5 total minutes of exercise*. You don't have to believe these incredible numbers. But I think you will, once you get into Power-*of*-10 yourself.

One or Two Workouts per Week?

Power-*of*-10 is optimized to combine exercise and proper recovery so you get the full benefits working out once a week. I define once-a-week as a rest period that varies between 5 and 7 full days after each workout. The majority of my clients love to work out this way, and you can too. That said, many people simply prefer to do Power-*of*-10 twice a week. They generally do a shorter workout each time—3 to 4 exercise sets—and may exercise at a slightly lower level of intensity. Their actual exercise time can still add up to the same number of minutes per week, they just do it in two sessions instead of one, with 3 to 4 days rest in between. Either way, you can end up with the same results. It really comes down to your own time schedule and preference.

Beginners Should Start Twice a Week

As you'll see in Part II, working out twice a week is a great idea for beginners. It lets you start off gradually with lighter weights and more reps. It gives you added practice and requires less intensity. You'll know when you're ready to switch to once-a-week. Or you can simply stay with twice-a-week as long as you like.

Why I Like Machines

Even though Power-*of*-10 can be performed at home or with dumbbells, as I'll show you in Part Two, there are several reasons why using machines, found at any good fitness center, is the Tenth Commandment. Number one is safety. If you train with free weights until true failure, you won't be able to guarantee you can control the weight at the end of each set. That means you can drop weights on yourself or others, or seriously pull muscles trying not to. Machines are designed to eliminate this danger completely. Another key to machines is that modern cam designs facilitate more balanced resistance over a wider range of motion, so you receive a greater benefit.

So, Once Again the 10 Commandments . . .

Here they are again—slightly abbreviated, but good to look at now that you've got some perspective. With these, and the specific exercises illustrated in full detail in Part II, you're ready to begin your first workout. This is Power-*of*-10 in 10 lines:

1 Thou Shalt Perform Repetitions of 10 Seconds Up, 10 Seconds Down.

2 Thou Shalt Not Hold Your Breath, but Shall Breathe Freely Throughout.

3 Thou Shalt Never Jerk the Weights Up or Down—Start Reps Smoothly.

4 Thou Shalt Do Reps Until Muscle Failure, Then Try for 10 More Seconds.

5 Thou Shalt Be Done in About 6 Individual Sets, If You Work Out Correctly.

6 Thou Shalt Choose a Weight, Allowing 8 Reps as a Beginner; 4 to 6 when Advanced.

7 Thou Shalt Move Quickly from Exercise to Exercise Until Done.

8 Thou Shalt Have a "Zen-like" Focus on Form, Speed, and Motion.

9 Thou Shalt Do One Workout per Week—Twice a Week, If You Feel Like It.

10 Thou Shalt Do Best and Be Safest If You Use Machines.

Now, Does Anyone Have Any Questions?

"Yes we do!" (Simulated response as if readers are bursting with questions):

- What about abs?

- What about stretching?

- What amount of aerobics is okay if I still like doing them?

- What if I'm a team athlete or do other strenuous sports?

- How long before I see real results?

- What if I don't belong to a gym?

- What if I want to work out dressed as Mary Ann from *Gilligan's Island*?

Almost all of these are great questions, deserving full answers; which appear in their own Q&A section at the end of Part I. Now, let's talk nutrition . . .

Steve Werner age 36

RETIRED NEW YORK CITY POLICE OFFICER

"You just can't believe it until you do it."

Weight lifting five days a week, 90 minutes at a time, finally caught up with me in November 1997. Or it caught up with my shoulders. I was a New York City cop who liked to stay in shape for my job physically and mentally with regular weight training. But here I was, recovering from my second blown-out shoulder, with the doctor telling me that

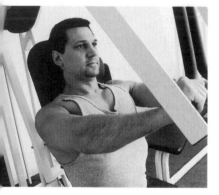

the weight training had to go or my job had to go because I'd end up disabled or worse. Almost every major upper body exercise depends on the shoulders. I'd been strong and athletic my whole life. Now I thought my life was over.

I was looking for something—anything—when a friend told me about Adam Zickerman and what he was doing with slow-cadence training. Above all, he said, it was safe. I called and scheduled a workout. After a few weeks of practice, Adam had me try chest and shoulder presses with Power-*of*-10. I was amazed that I could do them

without joint pain. I began regaining my lost strength. And within 6 weeks, incredible as it sounds, *all* my shoulder pain was gone! I was doing all the exercises that were supposedly taboo, getting stronger by the workout, waiting for the aches and pains to come—and they just never came. That was in 1998, and I've been pain free ever since. My life has changed in all kinds of ways since I started Power-*of*-10. Instead of practically living at the gym 5 days a week, I do my whole week's workout in one session, and I look better and feel better than before. I actually have time for a life outside the gym. My back was another thing that always bothered me from lugging weights around the gym every week, but today my back feels great. I actually got my body fat down to 8 percent *without cardio* at all—just Power-*of*-10 once a week.

Now I want you to know my saga's not quite finished. In 1999, I was chasing a suspect into the subway when my foot went through a broken stair and I tore apart my knee. That injury forced me to retire from the force. I've had three knee operations since.

But once again, I've rehabilitated myself with Power-*of*-10. I can walk distances now with little pain. My quads and hamstrings have regained much of their strength. I don't know what I would have done without the Power-of-10 protocols.

I would tell anyone at any age to embrace this exercise. You get the best workout in the world in a fraction of the time. You just can't believe it until you do it.

Exercise that can transform a body in about 20 minutes a week is not a miracle, but it's almost a miracle. To reach *miracle*, Pillar 1 needs Pillar 2. Great exercise needs great nutrition. From your first Power-*of*-10 workout, your recharging body will beg and beseech you for muscle-making, fat-foiling, cell-celebrating nutrients like never in your life. It will suck them up like a sponge all day, every

NUTRITION— THE 2ND PILLAR

day, so that it can do the powerful work you've unleashed it to do. It's simple: give your body the nutrition it needs and it'll give you your miracle.

TWO BIG IDEAS, ONE RULE

Power-*of*-10 Nutrition is based on the following two ideas plus a single rule. First, to build a magnificent body with lean muscle, you can't constantly give it food that generates fat. You feed it the food that generates lean muscle. As often as possible. What I'm going to ask you to do in this chapter is to trade the fat-making foods—sugar-filled soda pop, nachos and cheese; supersized fries, and monster cookies—for healthy muscle- and cell-making foods like delicious proteins, healthy fats, whole foods, and fiber.

Emphasis on delicious. I don't mean you can never have a Ben & Jerry's or a Snickers bar or real salad dressing, because you can. Just train your attention on the good stuff. It's how Olympic athletes, animals, primitive humans, movie stars, and Power-*of*-10 success stories eat.

Second, you don't get the benefits of great nutrition if it's so hard, time-consuming, and boring that you don't do it. Gee, where have I heard that before? A nutrition philosophy must be simple to follow, give the least sense of sacrifice, and allow real flexibility. Here again, Power-*of*-10 Nutrition is the best we've ever experienced.

Okay, that's the two big ideas. Now here's the rule:

Never diet.

D-I-E-T IS A "FOUR LETTER WORD"

I'm not trying to be coy, but Power-*of*-10 Nutrition is absolutely not and never will be a . . . I can't even say it—the "D word." You've probably heard this from other nutritionists, but it's not marketing spin and here's why. The moment you go on, all right, a *diet*, you go on a program that is psychologically tagged with denial, sacrifice, and restriction and is thus preset to fail from the beginning. Diets are temporary by definition, designed to be quit the minute you reach your weight loss goal. You hang on daily with the end in mind. When you get there, you stop on a dime and reward yourself with all the stuff you've been holding off like the enemy at the gates. In the process, since you've triggered your body's starvation response (which I'll talk about later), you've tuned yourself metabolically to gain back all the fat you've lost, plus even more, within a matter of days. You're worse off than when you started. Two or three months later when you've had enough time to grieve over your latest personal failure and have found some "closure," you go at it again. Now repeat the above paragraph.

Power-*of*-10 Nutrition is different because it's not a diet, it's a *way of living*. A way of fueling our bodies with the nutrition of champions every day. It's not about denying ourselves the foods that taste so good but make us fat, it's about knowing, wanting, loving—and therefore choosing the thousands of different kinds of foods that make us healthy, lean, and strong. You rarely miss the foods you choose not to have, because you think instead about all the scrumptious, wonderful foods that you *can* have. And with Power-*of*-10 Nutrition, if Mrs. Rumpworth hands you a piece of her cheesecake at the company picnic and it looks good, go ahead—enjoy it and move onward. You can't fail a way of living, as long as you don't quit.

THE MAIN REASON AMERICANS ARE SO FAT

When according to government statistics, 50 percent of a nation of 300 million people is officially obese or significantly overweight, I'm sorry, but something is out of control. We're dealing with a massive public health problem that annually costs us billions, not to mention the shortened, illness-ridden, physically curtailed lives suffered by these individuals. The rate of obesity has almost doubled in the last 25 years. Yet studies suggest we're not suddenly eating so much more, nor are we ingesting so much more fat, or exercising so much less to account for this crisis. What's happened is that little by little, convenience store by convenience store, TV commercial by TV commercial, our food culture has been transformed so that today Americans are literally swimming in a sea of sugar. Refined white sugar, high fructose corn syrup, dextrose, maltose, lactose, sorbitol, xylitol, to name a few. Fancy names, all sugar. They're the major ingredients in almost all the processed foods we eat, from canned soup to coleslaw. And "added sugar" isn't the only problem here, folks. The mountains of refined "starchy" carbohydrates we eat, from chips to snacks to crackers to giant servings of pasta and white flour breads, might as well be sugar because within minutes of entering your body, these carbohydrates metabolize into, guess what? Sugar. Add to that all the new "fat-free" processed foods, which replace the fat with more sugars and "white," processed carbohydrates, and you get a sense of the magnitude of it all. These ingredients insidiously generate more fat than if the fats had been kept in.

Why does sugar matter? Because the sugar we eat doesn't promote the growth of lean muscle, nerve, or cell tissue. Sugar is a "food" uniquely designed to turn into fat. It provides a huge number of calories devoid of the essential nutrients that could make it productive. Because it doesn't carry its own nutrients, it actually robs other vital nutrients from our bodies so it can be processed, further depleting our systems. And its constant presence leads to chronically high levels of insulin in the blood in order to control it. Insulin does many things. It regulates blood sugar. It helps transport nutrients to the cells—and it tells the body to store fat! No matter what you do, it's virtually impossible to lose weight when you're walking around with a chronically elevated insulin level the way so many Americans do.

I've gone on this sugar diatribe because sugar is the stealthy saboteur of so many people's efforts to get and stay fit. I also want you mentally prepared for the moment, just pages away, when I officially ask you to cut down on your chocolate chip cookie intake. The human body—designed over millions of years to eat protein, whole grains, leafy plants, fruits, and fiber—was never meant to ingest the current 145 pounds of sugar per year that's become the norm in the last hundred. We're paying an enormous physical toll for eating this way. Power-*of*-10 Nutrition solves the problem.

THE KEYS TO POWER-*OF*-10 NUTRITION

All food falls into one of three groups: protein, fat, and carbohydrates. All three are essential to sustain life. In today's food culture, it's the balance and quality of these three that have gotten completely out of whack. Power-*of*-10 Nutrition restores the balance and boosts the quality by default. I'll start you off by giving you a 30-second version for a quick perspective. Then I'll illustrate with details, strategies, and hints so you can get going on your own.

WHY IT'S SO EASY TO FOLLOW

You'll quickly see that 98 percent of the time, the foods you want to eat or avoid can be determined just by looking at them. Example: "See that buffet? Eat the turkey breast and the roast beef, the salad and the veggies, a little dressing on the side. Don't eat the bread sticks and the donut." There's no carrying around books, scales, or calculators. When you have a question, I'll show you how to read the labels. When I say "portion," I mean an amount about the size of a deck of cards.

POWER-*OF*-10 NUTRITION: 30-SECOND VERSION

- It helps for you to think of sugar as poison. Don't eat it.
- All the starchy "white things," like white flour, white rice, and potatoes, equal sugar.
- All junk-food snacks are made from 1 and 2 above.
- Eat a portion of lean protein with every meal and snack.
- Eat plenty of green and leafy vegetables and plenty (20–50 grams) of fiber every day.
- Eat good fats, especially olive oil.

- Eat whole grain foods like whole wheat and multigrain breads.

- Eat 6 times a day.

- Drink 2 to 4 quarts of water a day.

- For sweets, eat the satisfying low-sugar, low-calorie desserts and sweets I'll tell you about later.

- Now that you're a member of America's fitness elite, you don't have to forget your roots. Cheat for one whole day each week and eat pizza, banana splits, or anything you want.

POWER-*OF*-10 NUTRITION: THE EXPANDED VERSION

What to Eat

1. CANCEL YOUR SUBSCRIPTION TO SUGAR. Again we start with our mantra: delete all white, starchy carbohydrates. Not just white sugar, but refined white flour products, white rice, cornstarch, and regular pasta (see Pasta Reality, later in this chapter). All these foods might as well be sugar because they convert immediately from starch to sugar in the body. Cut way down on white potatoes. Unlike white rice—which may be a staple for two billion people, but has almost no nutrients besides starch—potatoes are packed with enough great nutrients to make them worthwhile. But remember, they still contain a lot of sugar-producing starch, so eat them very sparingly. And put absolute trace amounts of butter, fat, or sauces on top when you do.

Next, read the labels on processed foods. When you see sugar or the disguised sugar names like high fructose corn syrup, maltose, dextrose, xylitol, sorbitol, etc., early in the list, you know sugar's a main ingredient. Also, check the number of sugar grams on the label. Four grams of sugar equal 1 teaspoon. It adds up fast. A 12-ounce soda with 40 grams of sugar contains 10 *teaspoons*. Imagine that! You'll save 40 *teaspoons of sugar* just by switching from four regular sodas a day to diet soda! Sweeten foods with a sugar substitute like the new Splenda, which is now available. Splenda is a natural sugar derivative called sucralose without the bad properties of sugar, so it may taste more natural to you than aspartame or saccharin (Equal and Sweet 'n Low). Sugars that are not added, but occur naturally in things like whole fruits and dairy are generally okay. But be very careful of fruit juices—even the "no sugar added, 100% juice" kind. If you look at the label, you'll see the juice still contains a high, concentrated dose of sugar in the form of fructose, relative to fiber and other nutrients. If you're thirsty, water is always better.

2. EAT A PORTION OF LEAN PROTEIN IN EVERY MEAL OR SNACK. The essential amino acids in protein are the building blocks of lean muscle and the building blocks of life. I want you to eat more protein than you're used to—one portion in at least four of the six total meals and snacks you eat each day. I'll give you a more extensive list later, but lean proteins are white meat chicken, turkey breast, lean beef, lean pork, fish, shellfish, eggs, and low-fat cottage cheese, which is one of the most complete proteins of all. Another wonderfully convenient source is called whey protein powder. It's the main ingredient in high-quality meal replacement shakes, protein shakes, and protein bars you can find at any vitamin store, health food store, fitness center, and now in big supermarkets and pharmacies. Many nutritionists consider whey protein to be the best overall source of protein there is. Personally, because they're so convenient, I drink these shakes for two, sometimes three out of my six meals each day. As a rule of thumb, read the label and pick the ones that contain less than 5 grams of sugar and 5 grams of carbs. Likewise, pick meal replacement bars that have a ratio of at least one-third protein grams to total grams by weight, and contain less than 5 grams of sugar and less than 10 grams of carbs. Last but not least, in the Forty of My Favorite Snacks section, I'll show you easy ways to get protein into all your snacks, everything from slicing hard-boiled eggs on top of a small salad, to dropping a scoop of whey protein powder onto a bowl of cereal.

3. EAT PLENTY OF "DARK GREEN, RED, AND YELLOW THINGS": GREEN LEAFY AND CRUCIFEROUS VEGETABLES, AND FRUIT. Vegetables and whole fruits are the definition of great, essential carbohydrates. They provide vitamins, minerals, and added substances that scientists seem to discover every day, like antioxidants and phytochemicals, which ward off diseases like cancer and heart disease. They are an essential fuel for brain function. And they are a primary, natural source of the daily fiber you need to slow your body's production of insulin, to facilitate digestion, and to aid in the metabolizing of proteins. Green leafy vegetables include spinach, dark salad greens, kale, chard, and parsley. Cruciferous vegetables are things like broccoli, cauliflower, cabbage, and Brussels sprouts. And don't forget green beans, peas (technically a legume), asparagus, and more. A full list of fruits and vegetables is on page 42. You'll notice that some old stand-bys may not be on the list, such as corn, carrots, watermelon, and others. These have such a high starch or sugar content, you can easily avoid them without missing out on good health. It's hard to eat too many vegetables and whole fruit—and easy to eat too little. So, every day, I want you to eat vegetables and fruits with as many of your six meals and snacks as you can. It can be tougher to do this when you're eating out because traditional eating establishments place such a low emphasis on veggies. But don't give up, and no excuses. Get your delicious vegetables—no fewer than 3 portions per day.

4. BALANCE YOUR MEALS WITH WHOLE FOODS SUCH AS WHOLE GRAINS, BEANS, OR LEGUMES EACH DAY. The modern American food industry has done a marvelous job of increasing product shelf life; finding cheap, pleasant-tasting filler ingredients; and robbing most foods of all their essential food value by refining out the fiber, bran, husks, and skins where the nutrients are. All you have to do to get them back is to eat whole foods like whole grain breads, cereals, pastas, brown or wild rice, beans, and legumes, if you can, each day. A legume is pretty much any bean or pea, meaning everything from lentils, black beans, red kidney beans, and chickpeas (just eat hummus), to regular and split peas. Like most whole foods, these are a terrific source of vitamins, minerals, fiber, some protein—and the beneficial, low-sugar–producing carbohydrates—plus all the essential substances I'm sure scientists don't even know about yet. Getting your whole foods is quite simple. Just look at the label and make sure it says "whole grain." For example, real whole wheat bread will make sure you don't miss that fact by calling itself "100% stone-ground, whole wheat." Rye is also an excellent whole grain.

5. FIND WAYS TO EAT EXTRA FIBER EVERY DAY. Fiber ain't just for constipation any-more. It turns out it's essential for everything from proper digestion to disease fighting to getting that full feeling so you will eat less. And here's the big bonus—as fiber digests, it breaks down into acids that trigger the fat-burning process. Fiber, in combination with protein, makes up a muscle-building, fat-burning dynamic duo. Most of us need much more fiber than we get. Even if we eat whole foods, fruits, and vegetables each day, it's unlikely we're getting the 30 or more grams that are recommended, *minimum!* The eas-iest way to guarantee you take in enough fiber is to supplement at meals or snack times either by eating super-high-fiber cereal like Fiber One or All Bran, which can practically give your daily fiber allotment in a single bowl, or by adding powdered psyllium husk to water or juice, protein shakes, yogurt, etc. You can find powdered psyllium at any health food store and most supermarkets and pharmacies.

6. EAT SOME "GOOD" FATS EVERY DAY. Here's the story on fats. You can't live without them. Fats are crucial to brain, nerve, and general cell function. You don't need more than a few tablespoons per day—but you need fat. The trick is to eat the "good," unsaturated fats and only if you must. Eat tiny amounts of "bad," saturated fats or none at all. Good fats are naturally occurring fats that haven't been damaged by food processing. My all-time favorite is extra virgin olive oil because it's so easy to find, inexpensive, and tastes great with virtually everything. I use it in dressings and sauces, when I sauté, and in place of butter on whole wheat breads—just as the best restaurants do. The other good fats are found in virtually all fish, nuts, and avocados—my personal favorite food. Real fresh butter is even okay in small amounts. Here are your enemy fats: "trans-fats" like margarine, partially hydrogenated oils, and those fats found in all nonlean protein such as dark-meat poultry, fatty beef products, and pork products like bacon, hot dogs and sausage, and most organ meats.

7. DRINK 12 GLASSES OF WATER A DAY. I know you won't drink all 12, but maybe you'll drink 8. You're probably sick of hearing everybody tell you about water, but that's because every expert agrees it's vital to healthy cell function, muscle growth, elimination of body toxins and, especially, the efficient metabolizing of fat. It suppresses your appetite by filling you up. It improves the look of your skin. When you first start drinking water, you will find yourself in the bathroom more, but you'll adjust, especially if you spread your intake throughout the day. Now that you've got the water lecture, let me give you a hint that is heresy to most purists but better than not drinking enough if you just can't get yourself to down all that H_2O each day. Other liquids that are mostly water—from skim milk to juices to diet soft drinks to caffeinated coffee, believe it or not—will contribute to your water intake. Even though coffee's a diuretic, which means it causes you to eliminate water, you'll eliminate less than you'll keep. So don't get me wrong, water's by far the healthiest liquid. Short of that, hydrate yourself with any no-sugar-added, water-based fluid, and you're way better off than not drinking at all.

8. FLAVORING FOODS. Eating everything steamed is bo-ring! And I know from experience that an eating philosophy that bores you to death won't be around for long. So let yourself flavor things with *small amounts* of real butter, gravies, sauces, dressings—just have them on the side, especially if they contain sugar, flour, or saturated fats. It's one of the bonuses you get from cutting out all the sugar. Your body will be metabolizing fat so well, it can handle this tiny indulgence. And don't forget, things like salsa, horseradish, mustard, and soy sauce are great additions that carry no penalty at all.

9. TAKE A MULTIVITAMIN EVERY DAY. This is a no-brainer supplement. Even when we do our best to eat whole foods these days—natural vitamins and minerals have a way of losing their potency through cooking, processing, and long shelf lives. Taking a multivitamin daily virtually assures you'll make up the difference—enhancing cell function, supporting the immune system, and helping guard against disease.

How to Eat

10. NEVER SKIP MEALS OR LET YOURSELF GET HUNGRY. Hunger triggers the body's "starvation response" and slows your fat-burning metabolism to a stop. If you let yourself get hungry, you're not eating enough. Over eons of evolution, before supermarkets were even invented, our bodies developed a basic defense mechanism to deal with famine or the inconsistent availability of food. When we get hungry, our body decides to slow metabolism down to a crawl to avoid starvation. That means fat gets protected at all costs. This is the biggest irony for people who try to reduce their calories to a minuscule amount when they diet. Their state of constant hunger sabotages their efforts. And, cruelest of all, when they resume eating regular portions again, their superefficient metabolism accumulates fat like crazy, causing them to blow up like a balloon just by eating normally. You must eat enough never to be hungry. The answer is not to eat less food, but to eat more of the right food. This leads us to the next important point.

11. EAT SIX TIMES A DAY, ONCE EVERY 2 TO 3 HOURS, TO BURN EVERYTHING UP AS YOU GO. Think of this as three balanced meals around normal breakfast, lunch, and dinner times, with three balanced snacks in between. All six meals and snacks include at least a portion of lean protein. At *least three* of the six include a portion of vegetables. At *least two* of the six should include supplemental fiber sources. And at *least two* of the six should include other whole foods like whole grains, beans, or legumes. If you're just not hungry, skip the snacks, not the meals. But don't go more than three hours without eating something to avoid the starvation response. Because you'll be eating so often, it makes sense that the size of your meals should always be small to moderate. That's why I recommend the following portion sizes as a guide.

12. COUNT PORTIONS AT EACH MEAL, NOT CALORIES. A portion is the size of a deck of cards—about 20 grams. A balanced meal should be 3 to 4 portions. A balanced snack should be 2 portions. For example, a meal could be 1 or 2 portions of protein, a portion of vegetables, and a portion of brown rice or a slice of whole wheat bread, depending on how hungry you are. A snack can be a portion of low-fat cottage cheese and an apple, or a tablespoon of all-natural peanut butter on a slice of whole wheat bread.

13. ONCE A WEEK TAKE A FREE DAY AND EAT WHATEVER YOU FEEL LIKE. I mean cheesecake and a pile of fried rice if you want it. If you limit yourself to 1 day, your body will blow right by it without noticing. And the good news is, after a short time you'll lose your cravings for most of those foods anyway. You'll eat that chocolate chip cookie and realize it just isn't that good. Having your new lean body is so much better.

What to Eat for Dessert

I love sweet things, especially after spicy things. I would never give up sweets and neither should you. There are hundreds of ways to "have your cake and eat it too"—they just don't involve New York cheesecake or caramel crème brûlée, except on your off-day or birthday. In a calorie-free world, my first choice would be a big brownie with Häagen-Dazs Dulce de Leche and hot fudge every time. But in *this* world, I pick mixed berries with a scoop of delicious, sugar-free vanilla ice cream; or scores of other choices I'll give you. Because with these choices, I get gratified two for one: I get a sweet taste delight, plus I get to leave the table with my lean fit body intact. And that's a great deal.

There are so many ways to get your sweet fix—and we all know that fresh fruits are the healthiest. But I'm not such a goody-goody that I'd try to sell you on a bowl of fruit as a substitute for an ice cream sundae. Far from it. You can take that fruit, mix it with low-fat vanilla yogurt or sugar-free ice cream, which is surprisingly good, and make a huge smoothie milk shake that's to die for. Or eat any of the dozens of varieties of low-fat, sugar-free frozen bars and treats like Creamsicles, Fudgsicles, fruit juice bars, and ice cream sticks. There're more and more to choose from every day because so many of us now are into the low-sugar, low-carb way of living, and food corporations are responding.

TIPS ON MAKING BALANCED MEALS AND SNACKS

Until the day when every Quik-Stop Convenience Mart is dedicated to lean protein and whole foods, I know there are going to be times when you can't put together the perfect protein-fat-carbohydrate combo for every one of your meals and snacks. Doesn't matter. You'll succeed just by keeping your goal in mind and sincerely trying. It's easiest at home. Just make sure you've stocked up on items from the balanced food lists on page 42—the proteins, vegetables, grain products, legumes, etc. Then just fix yourself a portion of each and you've got a meal. Do the same for snacks. But since you're usually eating those on the run, or may want a little variety because, let's face it, turkey breast with coleslaw doesn't really sound like a snack, I've included forty of my favorite snacks.

Eating out is just a little harder. All I can say is, you'll get better at improvising and making good choices with practice. And there are going to be times, like at the business conference when the continental breakfast is all donuts and Danish, that you're going to be stuck with a cup of coffee until you can get to the restaurant. That's one reason why I always carry a couple of quality meal replacement protein bars in my briefcase.

GOOD FOODS

The following is a partial list of the kinds of foods I've been talking about. To make a balanced meal, all you do is pick a portion of protein, then pick one or two items from the other lists. The more vegetables, fruits, and legumes the better. Keep the breads and whole grain products down to 2 portions per day.

GOOD LEAN PROTEINS

Chicken breast

Turkey breast

Lean ground beef

Lean trimmed beef

Lean trimmed lamb

Ham

Trimmed pork

Trimmed veal

Game birds

Crab

Fish of all kinds

Lobster

Shrimp

Shellfish like clams, oysters, and mussels

Eggs

Low-fat cottage cheese

Whey protein

Tofu

GOOD VEGETABLES

Artichokes

Broccoli

Cabbage

Cauliflower

Celery

Cilantro

Eggplant

Garlic

Ginger

Green beans

Leafy salad greens

Lentils

Mushrooms

Okra

Onions

Parsley

Peas

Peppers

Spinach

Squash

Zucchini

GOOD FRUITS

Apples

Apricots

Avocados

Berries of all kinds

Cantaloupes

Cherries

Cucumber

Figs

Grapes

Honeydew melon

Kiwis

Lemons

Limes

Nectarines

Oranges

Peaches

Pears

Plums

Strawberries

Tangerines

Tomatoes

GOOD BEANS AND LEGUMES

Black beans

Chick peas

Fava beans

Kidney beans

Lentils

Lima beans

Navy beans

Peas

Pinto beans

Soybeans

GOOD RICES AND GRAIN PRODUCTS

Brown rice

Whole rice

Wild rice

Barley

Whole oats

Whole wheat

Whole grain pastas

GOOD FAT SOURCES

Canola oil

Flaxseed oil

Olive oil, extra virgin

Peanut oil

Fats found in all fish

Seeds

Pure butter in small amounts

THE GLYCEMIC INDEX: NATURAL WHOLE FOODS TO AVOID

Believe it or not, there are some whole fruits and vegetables that are so full of starch or convert to sugar so quickly, you can avoid them and be better off. The reason is something you'll run across in most modern weight-loss books, if you haven't already—a property of foods called the "Glycemic Index." It's a measurement not of how much sugar, but how *rapidly* different foods convert to sugar in the blood. The theory is that foods that turn instantly to sugar—such as the "white foods"—enter the bloodstream more quickly, causing the biggest insulin spikes and the most metabolic problems. On the other hand, foods that convert to sugar gradually allow the body to absorb it without an insulin bump and therefore don't trigger the fat storing response. Like all nutrition theories, the Glycemic Index is controversial. Some diet plans base their entire program around it; others dismiss it. I think it makes enough sense to say that the answer is somewhere in between. Therefore, I suggest you avoid the high glycemics just to be safe. There are so many other wonderful foods to choose from, you won't shortchange your body in any way.

The Glycemic Index is generally based on a scale of 100 to 1. White table sugar (sucrose) rates among the highest with a score of 100. The lowest scores are for green vegetables, which come in at 10 to 0. Based on the Glycemic Index, these are the vegetables and fruits you'd most want to avoid:

Beets	Potatoes (see Note)	Pineapple
Carrots	White rice	Raisins
Parsnips	Bananas (see Note)	Watermelon

NOTE: Yes (sigh), potatoes and bananas are high enough to be considered "white foods." But as I've mentioned previously, they're loaded with so many other nutrients, my advice is just to eat them very sparingly. I love bananas. A few slices thrown into a protein shake will never hurt. Neither will half a baked potato every now and then. *EVERY NOW AND THEN.* If you start having piles of mashed potatoes again with every dinner, I'll come to your house and take them away permanently. Potato chips and French fries are in the same category as cheesecake: off-day only.

But the Index Also Giveth . . .

Just so you're not completely distressed after learning about potatoes and bananas, you'll find the Glycemic Index doesn't just take tasty foods away, it also gives great foods back. The Index says it's okay to eat avocados and all-natural peanut butter, for example—two things we were always taught would turn us into an instant blimp. The good news is, they're all "good" fat and great sources of protein, vitamins, and minerals with a low Glycemic Index. So, go ahead and enjoy avocados and all-natural peanut butter—two of my favorite foods!

For a complete Glycemic Index listing of common foods, simply search on *glycemic index* in any Web search engine and you'll find glycemic values for all your favorites.

FINAL HINTS FROM THE REAL WORLD

1. Moderation in All Things. Except Vegetables

Common sense tells you that if you eat too much of anything, you won't lose fat. Keep the volume within reasonable bounds. And remember, Power-*of*-10 Nutrition is not a "high-fat/low-carb" diet where you can eat fat galore, as long as you cut out the sugar and carbs. If you eat volumes of saturated fat for the rest of your life, you'll end up dead of heart disease, making it much harder to attract members of the opposite sex. Fried foods, bacon, sausage—all the classic heavy, fatty things—are to be eaten in extreme moderation. You will be a *much* healthier, better-looking person.

2. Calories Count—It's Just That No One Succeeds by Counting Calories

The old calorie theory of weight control is still true. If you burn more calories than you take in, you lose weight. Calorie counting is just the most tedious, complicated and most guaranteed-to-be-given-up method of nutrition planning I know. Glycemic Index and unhealthy fats aside, a great thing that happens with Power-*of*-10 Nutrition is that we're automatically slashing our calorie consumption while increasing our ratio of quality, lean muscle-producing nutrients, simply by substituting all the good stuff for huge volumes of sugar, white carbs, and saturated fats. You're saving a mountain of calories by replacing a pile of pasta, Alfredo sauce, and three large cookies with a Dijon chicken breast, spinach sautéed in olive oil, a sweet potato, and berries with yogurt for dessert. And every bite makes you happy because you know you're eating the ingredients that foster lean muscle, not fat.

3. Pasta Reality

I know many of you hate me for telling you to say farewell to the love of your life: regular white pasta. But if you think about it, it's only in the last twenty years that Americans have gotten used to eating monster plates of pasta at practically every meal. It seems like everything from crab cakes to Jell-O is served on a "bed of pasta." Add to that the high-calorie sauces and toppings that normally go with it, and you can picture the old movie *Requiem for a Heavyweight* with you as the heavyweight. Look, I love pasta as much as you do. So let me suggest this: while you're in your maximum fat-shrinking mode, really try to cut pasta out, except of course on your off-day. You'll save a ton of calories and converted sugar. Then, when you get to your goal of weight and trimness, eat a little portion now and then, that's all. Just change the habit of eating a giant plate of pasta as a main meal 3 to 4 times a week. And don't forget, whole grain pasta is delicious and qualifies as a whole grain food.

4. A Label Says a Thousand Words

Ninety-five percent of the foods you'll either eat or avoid with Power-*of*-10 Nutrition don't have and don't need labels. Whole foods like chicken, cabbage, and brown rice don't have labels. And you don't need the label on a shrink-wrapped pound of bacon for you to know it's a major source of the saturated fat you want to skip.

When it comes to processed foods, from canned sauce to breakfast cereal, you'll want to check the label to see what's really in them. The main thing you should know is that ingredients are listed in order from greatest to least amounts in the product. So when you see that one of the top three ingredients is any of the sugars mentioned earlier—from regular sugar to high fructose corn syrup, dextrose, maltose, lactose, sucrose, sorbitol, xylitol, or any of the other alcohols that end in "itol"—you know what you're dealing with. With respect to genuine whole grain flour instead of white refined flour,

Nutrition Facts	Amount/Serving	%DV**	Amount/Serving	%DV**
Serving Size 1 pack	**Total Fat** 13g	20%	**Total Carb.** 30g	10%
	Sat. Fat 5g	25%	Fiber 2g	8%
Calories 250	**Cholest.** 5mg	2%	Sugars 25g	
Fat Calories 120	**Sodium** 25mg	1%	**Protein** 5g	
** Percent Daily Values (DV) are based on a 2,000 calorie diet.	Vitamin A*	Vitamin C*	Calcium 4%	Iron 2%
	Thiamin 2%	Riboflavin 4%	Niacin 8%	
	* Contains less than 2 percent of the Daily Value of these nutrients.			

INGREDIENTS: MILK CHOCOLATE (SUGAR, CHOCOLATE, COCOA BUTTER, SKIM MILK, LACTOSE, MILKFAT, PEANUTS, SOY LECITHIN, SALT, ARTIFICIAL FLAVORS), SUGAR, PEANUTS, CORNSTARCH, LESS THAN 1% CORN SYRUP, GUM ACACIA, COLORING (INCLUDES RED 40 LAKE, BLUE 2 LAKE, BLUE 1 LAKE, YELLOW 6, YELLOW 5, RED 40, BLUE 1, BLUE 2, YELLOW 5 LAKE, YELLOW 6 LAKE), DEXTRIN.

YOU CAN'T HAVE THIS! A nutrition label from a typical chocolate bar.

the manufacturers really spell it out. You'll see something like, "100% Stone-Ground Whole Wheat" versus enriched or fortified wheat flour in the ingredients list. "Enriched" is a big red flag. It means they took all the natural goodness out during processing, then they put a little back in. "Fortified" means they added some nutrient to make it more healthful. The nutritional breakdown on the label is also pretty straightforward. Four grams of sugar per serving equals 1 teaspoon. When I'm checking breakfast cereals, it's easy to compare them by sugar content. Some have 20 grams per serving. Others have none. "No added sugar" products may still have sugars—but they're natural and are much better than the refined kind. The natural sugar products generally have a low Glycemic Index as well. So, don't fret unnecessarily when you see them. A cup of skim milk has 12 grams of natural milk sugar, for example, and a Glycemic Index of only 30 (out of 100). A cup of tomato juice has 8 grams of natural sugar and a Glycemic Index of only 15. You can certainly drink them. Finally, expect to see 20 to 30 grams of "carbohydrates" listed on such products as whole wheat bread or whole grain cereals. After all, that's what they are: carbohydrates. You're supposed to be eating carbs when you eat these things. Just eat them in moderation.

5. Dodging Refined White Flour

This one's simple. All commercial baked goods contain it, unless it's specifically listed as 100 percent whole grain. That means bagels, donuts, cookies, cakes, pitas, pizza dough, pies, muffins, tortilla wraps—everything. And unless they say "sugar free" the sweet taste always comes from some form of sugar.

6. If You Really Can't Resist, Take One Bite

Trust me, it's actually easier to take no bites. "Out of mouth, out of mind."

7. Measuring Your Progress: It's About Losing Fat, Not Pounds

Some nutritionists happily shout, "Throw out your scale." I can only say, if you did that where I live, you'd probably hit someone on the sidewalk and get arrested. The fact is, the scales has its place. Your total weight will and should go down over the weeks and months as you get more and more fit, unless you're starting Power-*of*-10 with very low body fat. It's satisfying to see. Just know that the scale has so many off-setting factors, you'll needlessly distress yourself if you weigh yourself every single day. You can vary 5 pounds a day in water weight; several pounds if you ate a late dinner. If you're gaining pounds of lean muscle while losing fat like you should, your weight on the scale won't drop as much, even though your waistline and measurements are shrinking. Unless you're a boxer trying to make a weight class, what this is really all about is losing fat, not losing a weight number. Pinching your sides every night in bed and feeling the fold get tighter is every bit as good as getting on a scale, maybe better. I still have this one belt that gives me a 32-inch waist on the third hole. When the belt gets a little tighter, I tighten the screws for a few days and maybe skip the small portions of bread and pasta. My belt's the best gauge I know. I also keep my scale, however, and check it now and then, just to give me another benchmark. Using a scale or not is up to you—just use it intelligently.

8. Drinking Alcohol

Alcohol is fattening. About 150 calories a shot. That said, for the average adult, one shot of alcohol per day is considered to have more therapeutic benefits than drawbacks for preventing heart disease, stress related problems, even cancer. If you're over twenty-one, one drink a day is absolutely fine. Most experts think red wine is your best choice. If you love beer, choose a light beer, because beer in general is high on the Glycemic Index. Just know that anything over one shot quickly switches to the negative side of the nutritional balance sheet.

8. How About Cheese and Dairy Products?

Cheese is a good source of protein, but *not* a lean protein. Most cheeses are also high in saturated fat and contain about 100 calories per ounce—that's a cube that measures about ¾ inch by ¾ inch. Be moderate with cheese. Use low-fat or no-fat dairy products whenever possible. Nutritionists have been arguing for years about the pluses and minuses of dairy consumption for adults. If you're not lactose intolerant and can digest it properly, again select the lowest-fat dairy product you can find, and eat it in moderation.

9. People Who Succeed Plan and Think About It a Little Every Day

One of the best things I ever read was an article about a recent study on people who succeed at fitness. It found that the concept of someone dieting for a while, losing all the weight, then trying to stop dieting and relax once they reach their goal is an utter myth. The only adults over age twenty who really stay trim, fit, and young-looking into middle age and beyond are those who think and plan their nutrition and their fitness program a little each day—every day. They think ahead about what they're going to eat. If they overdo a meal or two, they cut back for a few meals to make up for it. They think about how and where and when they're going to get in their workouts. It's a lifelong process, folks. If you want it, you invest the little bit of time and energy it takes to get it. It's a permanent priority. But it pays you back in spades. And because it's so satisfying to be fit and strong and youthful at any age, it becomes easy to make it a habit for life.

FINALLY—IF BEING BUFF, HEALTHY, STRONG, ENERGETIC, AND THE IDOL OF EVERYONE AT YOUR HIGH SCHOOL REUNION ISN'T MOTIVATION ENOUGH—A LITTLE GUILT HELPS

Okay, when it's not your off-day, be my guest and feel a little guilty if you down an entire wheel of Brie at your aunt's house. There are so many great things riding on your ability to make good nutrition choices, you should feel a tad negative if you start letting yourself down. Not for a bite here and there, but if you really get lax. If guilt's what it takes, don't knock it. After all, if you're Catholic or Jewish, you know that guilt powers the world. The fact is, I don't think you're going to need it. There is no feeling in the world like being in the best shape of your life. Pillar 1 and Pillar 2 will transport you to fitness like the Yellow Brick Road to the Emerald City. Remember, all you do is follow it and pay homage to the third and final Pillar along the way . . .

ONE MO' TIME

- Stop eating sugar.

- Stop eating the other "white things."

- Eat lean protein each time you eat.

- Eat plenty of the "dark green, red, and yellow things."

- Eat extra fiber every day.

- Eat a little of the "good" fats like olive oil; don't eat the "bad" saturated fats.

- Eat whole foods.

- Eat moderate-size meals and snacks, 6 times a day.

- Drink tons of water.

- Eat low-calorie, nonsugar sweets and desserts.

- Take one day off a week and eat anything you want.

Malena Belafonte

PROFESSIONAL FASHION MODEL, SINGER, ACTRESS

How a Successful Model Simplified Her Life . . .

Obviously I have to stay in shape for the work I do. The problem was that my routine required 4 to 5 workouts a week at the gym, doing free weights, definition classes, yoga, and spinning. Time always seemed to be working against me. I never know where I'm going to be from one day to the next, or what my shoot-ing schedule is going to be. So while I enjoyed working out, the stress of just trying to fit the time in sometimes made it seem more distressing than it was worth. I'd feel as though I'd let myself down if I skipped the gym. Miss 3 days in a row and I'd really feel guilty.

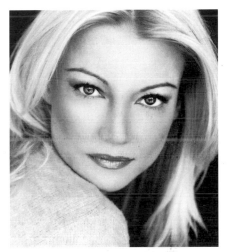

About a year ago, I just happened to read about Adam's exercise techniques in *Newsweek*. Intuitively, it just seemed to make sense that going slow would have a deeper effect and the promise of cutting workouts down to once or twice a week was so appealing, I decided to test the concept for myself.

What I liked immediately was the sense of focus that's part of the program. I found it challenging and refreshing. My muscles felt like they'd been thoroughly worked out in so few exercises. To get that same feeling of satisfaction from a workout would normally take me much longer. Within the first 2 weeks, I actually started to see more definition in my arms and shoulders, and began feeling stronger. I felt that Adam's philosophy was perfectly suited to me. I even began applying the focus of Power-*of*-10 to other aspects of my life. If problems seem too overwhelming, I know how to take a step back, breathe, focus on the problem at hand, and go for it.

I still take my spinning, yoga, and other classes when I can because I do enjoy them. But if my schedule makes me miss them now, there's no stress and no problem. I know I'm getting my whole week of exercise in one or two 20-minute Power-*of*-10 workouts. So when I get to my spinning class, it's gravy.

Power-*of*-10 has taken a whole element of pressure out of my busy routine and I'm really grateful. It's a permanent part of my lifestyle. For me, it's about 20 minutes of exercise, once or twice a week. I think that's doable for just about anyone.

49

IT MAY BE THE MOST IMPORTANT PILLAR OF ALL

This is going to be a short but crucial chapter. I'll begin by paraphrasing a noted author and fitness expert:

Rest & Recovery is the one great pillar of fitness that most programs neglect—yet it's probably the biggest success secret of Power-of-10. In Power-of-10, we literally rest our way to success. Because rest, for

REST & RECOVERY —THE 3RD PILLAR

4

people trying to create fit, strong bodies, is as crucial as protein, oxygen, or any other nutrient. During exercise our muscle tissue breaks down and our bodies get temporarily weaker, not stronger. It's during rest that we recover and make all our gains. This is a huge, unspoken problem with even the most popular weight-training and exercise programs. When you are either at the gym lifting, or on the treadmill treading 6 days per week, you can't possibly have time for the rest your body needs. You're prone to muscle tears and strains, joint problems, chronic fatigue, and weakening of the immune system, so you get sick and get hurt more often . . . Power-of-10 is brilliantly designed to let you get the rest you need between workouts. Your rest is built-in.

Okay, I stole that from the Introduction to this book. But I did it to dramatize yet another way that Power-*of*-10 turns negatives into positives. The negative: I couldn't think of anything else to write. The positive: I took a lovely half-hour nap with the time I saved, providing an excellent example of Rest & Recovery.

HOW MUCH REST DO YOU REALLY NEED?

The exact amount of rest you need varies from person to person, just as some people do well on 7 hours of sleep a night while others need 9. Here's what I can say based on fitness research, years of training, and common sense: when you cause billions of microscopic tears in your muscle cells, as you do when you exercise thoroughly and properly, they don't recover 100 percent in 24 to 48 hours. Maybe it's enough when you're doing an inefficient conventional workout, throwing barbells around with no real intensity. But not when you're fatiguing all the cells as profoundly as you do in Power-*of*-10. It takes double that time to recover—about 4 days if you're doing the less intense, twice-a-week workouts, and 5 to 7 days when you're working out to full intensity, once a week. I even know some Power-*of*-10 people who find their optimum to be once every 9 days. In any case, I've never had a scrape or an abrasion that completely healed in 2 days, have you? It usually takes a week. And the older we get, the longer it takes for anything to heal and recover.

So, how do you find the off-period that's right for you? In the beginning, when you're working out twice a week, wait until the fourth day to work out again—even if you think you're feeling great and energetic after 2 or 3 days. Don't experiment until you've practiced enough to know you're doing the exercises right and reaching muscle failure each set. Then experiment a bit if you want to. Working out twice a week, you'll find you're optimum at between 3 and 5 days' rest.

When you switch to once a week, if you're like most people, your optimum layoff will be 5 to 7 full days. With practice, you'll know by keeping in tune with your body. If you are an experienced once-a-week person who tried to work out after only 4 days' rest, you would sense it immediately. You'd feel sluggish and weary during your workout, and you'd reach failure much more quickly. You'd know you needed another day or two of rest.

No matter what you do, never forget this rule: *Don't overtrain*. Power-*of*-10 exercise is so powerful and concentrated, you can quickly overdo it if you don't rest with the same level of commitment that you give to your workout. Rest like a champion. When in doubt with Power-*of*-10, less gives you more.

YOUR DAILY "HOUR OF POWER"

With Power-*of*-10, the time for you to rest is automatically built-in because you have nearly every day off. But let me make one thing perfectly clear: this rest is only there if you take it! In other words, don't use the golden opportunity you've received to add another hour of stress and aggravation to your life. Take that hour each day, when you'd be slugging it out at the gym, and think of it as your "hour of power." Pamper yourself with it, rejuvenate yourself with it, nourish yourself with it. This is no sissy, new age advice, folks. Quality rest is how people get big and strong. Think of it as real fitness time, because reduction of daily stress is a physical necessity if you want to ward off disease and stay healthy. When your body is stressed, it releases the hormone cortisol, among other stress hormones. Cortisol pumps up your heart rate, your breathing, and blood flow, because it's preparing you for fight-or-flight—the primitive response to danger. When you experience elevated cortisol levels on a regular basis, the effect can be devastating to health. Among other things, your blood pressure goes up, your immune system goes down, and digestion and sleep are adversely affected. So it's not a stretch to say that a little stress reduction each day can be significant to overall fitness.

Nowadays we have to actively plan our recovery and destressing time, just like we have to schedule any important activity. So make this a priority and do it for no other reason than, if you don't, I'll find out where you live, come to your house, and make you do sit-ups.

GREAT THINGS TO DO DURING YOUR HOUR OF POWER

The hour of power is about relaxing and destressing. In its purest form, that could mean taking an afternoon nap—one of the healthiest, most rejuvenating activities I know. During world crises, John F. Kennedy and Winston Churchill were famous for taking regular naps to recoup their energy. But really, any time you take out of the day for *you*, time that feels positive and nonstressful, will qualify. Paying your bills does not qualify, unless you just came into a fortune and you're actually having fun paying your credit cards down to zero. Here're some other suggestions.

Yoga and Stretching

The ancient practice of yoga is wildly popular these days for a reason. In my opinion, everything yoga does is good if you follow the principles of moderation I'll discuss in the Q&A section under "Pillar 1: Exercise." Yoga can increase strength, flexibility, and balance.

It increases blood flow to the muscles. It releases endorphins. It is incredibly soothing and relaxing. Yoga puts you in deep touch with your whole body and heightens your mental-physical connection. At the end of an hour session of yoga, you can feel like you've had a whole body massage and done an hour of transcendental meditation at the same time. It's energizing and therapeutic. The best way to start is to attend a class once or twice a week. They're generally inexpensive, and you can find them anywhere. With a little experience, you can practice anytime, anyplace.

Massage

If more people got a real therapeutic massage once a month, there would be no more war. Everyone would be too relaxed to care. Therapeutic massage is generally not something most people can afford more than once or twice a month. But its restorative and healing powers for muscle and mind are legendary. It will make 1 hour of power feel like 6.

Anything Else, from Meditation to Skydiving

The point should be clear by now. Anything that takes your mind or body off its stress track for an hour is a good thing. It could be reading romance novels in the tub or gardening or playing with the cat. It could be skydiving. I know several New York City cops who skydive every weekend because it's the one thing that completely frees their minds from the stuff they deal with every day on the job. Skydiving to them is 100 percent pure joy, beauty, and satisfaction—done with friends. For these guys, it relieves stress! Pick whatever turns you on or, more appropriately, what turns you off. Bestow it on yourself in your hour of power—one of the best fringe benefits of Power-*of*-10.

Sleep

There's no bigger priority in the recovery department than getting enough sleep. Most of us don't. The average person needs *at least* 8 hours of sleep a night, yet 43 percent of Americans say they usually sleep only 6 hours or less; and thus spend their lives chronically tired. Perhaps they wouldn't if they knew how important sleep is to health. When you're sleep deprived, your immune system suffers. You lose your ability to maintain focus and control your moods. Sleep deprivation has even been shown to impede weight loss because your body doesn't burn calories as efficiently.

Make a commitment to sleep 8 hours a night. It helps immensely to go to bed and wake up at the same time every day. Don't take stimulants like caffeine any time after 5 P.M. Don't ever drink alcohol to help you sleep. Alcohol produces a shallow, fitful sleep that will have you awakening in the middle of the night. When your body feels too tense to relax at bedtime, a few minutes of light stretching or even yoga can work wonders. And if you're really a problem sleeper, it's more than worth it to talk to a specialist. Your doctor can recommend one. Almost nothing will have a greater impact on your fitness, health, and well-being than getting adequate sleep—especially if you're one of the legions of walking sleep deprived. Start tonight.

THE 30-SECOND PILLAR 3

Pillar 3 is really that simple. The fact that Power-*of*-10 lets you devote 6 out of 7 days to rest makes it kind of a no-brainer and A PERSON WOULD HAVE TO BE AN IDIOT TO SCREW UP REST, WOULDN'T THEY! I'm sorry, I lost my head, but I get emotional when I think about people having all this extra time to relax and recover, and not taking full advantage of it. So here are the rules of Power-*of*-10 Rest & Recovery in a nutshell:

- Commit to rest the way you commit to exercise and nutrition.
- Rest 5 to 7 full days if working out once a week; 3 to 4 days if twice a week.
- Give yourself a free "hour of power" to relax and recover each day.
- Never overtrain. If your progress stalls, rest additional days.
- Get 8 hours sleep per night.

Now you've got all 3 Pillars and a new quality of life right within your grasp. After a bit of Q&A, we'll go on to Part II: The Power-*of*-10, Step-by-Step Workout. So let's . . . get ready . . . to RUM-MBLE! (always remembering to breathe and use proper form).

Barbara Murphy age 27

MOTORCYCLE ENTHUSIAST

To Ride Like the Wind, It Mattered What Shape She Was In . . .

People who don't ride motorcycles don't know how strenuous it can be, particularly if you're not in shape. My new Italian Ducati weighs 500 pounds. The more flexible and strong you are, the safer and more skilled you're going to be, especially when you get in a tight spot. And just having more energy and endurance makes riding more fun.

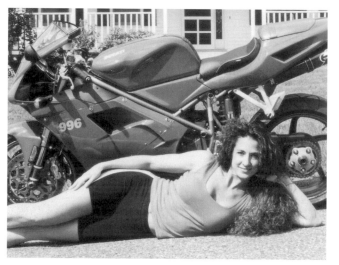

I started getting heavily into riding over a year ago, and I quickly realized I wasn't as strong as I used to be as a teen. I also started realizing that I couldn't eat whole boxes of Cheesy-Poofs anymore without consequences to my waistline. It was time to find a gym.

I did the round of the local fitness places. But they were all the same, selling me on multiple days of aerobics classes and weight training every week. None of them fit my crazy work or weekend schedule. And I couldn't stand the idea of living at the gym, anyway. So when my girlfriend told me about the Power-*of*-10 method, I had to give it a try. I wouldn't have believed the claims of once-a-week fitness, but she was doing it and getting great results. So I went for a session.

The first thing I noticed was that the slow intensity felt really great to me. I loved the focus and concentration. In 25 minutes, I was out of there, feeling like every single muscle in my body had been put through its paces. I also could understand how it could work in just 1 day a week. It felt like such deep exercise, I was glad to have the extra days off for rest and recovery. I wasn't really that sore afterward, but I could still feel that worked-out feeling a few days later.

I've become a regular now, and I can honestly say I love Power-*of*-10. I love the convenience and the feeling I get. Until they try it themselves, no one believes it. But once they try it, everyone does. I promise you one thing, you won't see a fatty on my Ducati!

The most common question about Power-*of*-10 isn't even asked, it's a *thought* people get when they hear about a program that's fully effective with 20 minutes of exercise, once a week.

The answer to this thought is, "No."

No, Power-*of*-10 will not give you miraculous, instant results without any effort. No, you can't accomplish your goals without a

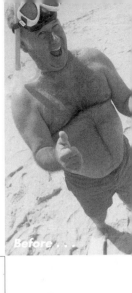

Before

QUESTIONS & ANSWERS

"I went from buffalo to buff in just two weeks!"

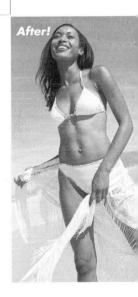

After!

serious commitment. No, you won't be transformed by magic like the "before and after" photos shown here. No, it's not something you do for a couple of months, get in shape, then stop and stay that way. Fitness forever is a way of life forever. Real programs like Power-*of*-10 take real resolve, real time, and have real up and down days. What I *am* promising you with Power-*of*-10 is a program designed to be as "quit-proof" as a fitness program can possibly be, because it's the easiest to follow, safest, most time-efficient fitness program you've ever found. And if you don't quit, you *will* succeed!

The following Q&A cover every other common question I've been asked over the years by beginners and experienced people alike. If any question remains after you read the ones here, e-mail me at my website at www.power-of-10.com, and I'll be sure to get back to you.

QUESTION & ANSWERS FOR PILLAR 1: EXERCISE

1. What About Abs?

There's a myth that abs are somehow different from other muscles, so it's okay to do them every day. Wrong. Abs are skeletal muscle like any other. Don't overtrain them. They should be exercised to failure, then allowed to rest and recover properly for best results. I've included several of my favorite abs exercises in Part Two. You'll also find that a great many of the compound exercises will effectively work abs as well. Bottom line: exercise your abs once or twice a week with the rest of your Power-*of*-10 program if you want to. Contrary to what commercials for TV abs gizmos might tell you—there's no such thing as "spot reducing," where you burn fat specifically in your middle by doing hundreds of abs crunches. The number one way to create a "six-pack" is through proper nutrition that reduces body fat over time. When you see someone with a six-pack, it's not so much built as it is *exposed*. They've stripped away the fat covering their abs and the rest of their body by eating properly, so you can see what's underneath.

2. What About Stretching?

Just like aerobics, many people in the fitness industry have made a kind of cult out of stretching, believing that it's the key to circulation, flexibility, muscle health, and even strength. My personal take on stretching is that if ever there was a place to apply the rule "moderation in all things," this is it. The fact is, you don't *need* to stretch if you do any form of resistance training that uses a full range of motion. With Power-*of*-10, just like its built-in warm-up, the stretching is *also* built-in. Every time you contract or flex one muscle, you automatically extend or stretch the opposing muscle. Flex your bicep at the front of your arm and you stretch the triceps in back. Your muscles will naturally move your joints through the range of motion that nature intended, without the risk of hyperextension or joint injury. And contrary to popular belief, muscles don't become tighter when they get stronger or become more elastic when stretched. Muscles become softer and more pliable through the increased blood flow that comes from strength training. The reality is, if you strength-train properly, extra stretching will not make you more healthy and fit, and excessive stretching can lead to a permanent elongation of the ligaments and the connective tissue that holds together the joints. Such joint laxity can cause significant injury over time. If you are a regular stretcher or yoga enthusiast, the best way to prevent joint laxity is by strengthening the muscles that surround and stabilize the joints through proper resistance training. So here's my bottom line: stretching can be pleasant and relaxing and restful. I certainly don't oppose it. Just be moderate. It's best to stretch *after* your workout when your muscles are warm. Never bounce when you stretch and never force your stretch past the point of pain. Back off any stretch if you feel discomfort. And listen to your body.

3. What Amount of Aerobics Is Okay If I Still Like Doing Them?

It depends on your fitness goals. If your goal is to build lean muscle mass as quickly and efficiently as possible, but you still enjoy aerobic exercise like walking or cycling, go ahead. Just do the exercises moderately. Whatever you do, it's always best to rest the day of your workout and a full day afterward, if you can. Then go ahead and do your aerobic exercises 2, 3, or 4 times during the week before your next workout. But instead of doing an hour or more of aerobics to full exhaustion, go easier—try 25 to 35 minutes instead. There's no exact science here. If you find you're plateauing out on your "Time Until Failure" (TUF) in certain sets, or even regressing, you may be overdoing the aerobics. Remember, you don't need to do aerobics to be completely fit with Power-*of*-10. The pressure to spend hours on the treadmill or bicycle each week is off. Do aerobics if they make you feel good, not if they're a chore.

4. What If I'm a Team Athlete or Engage in Other Strenuous Sports?

Here again, it depends on your priorities. If you're a college hockey player who skates 5 days a week to utter exhaustion, you can't do a full Power-*of*-10 workout in the middle of your schedule without overtraining. If possible, try to train on a day when you can take a day off afterward to recover. You may also find that you need more than a week's rest or a less intense workout. Try working out every 10 days, or doing 4 instead of 6 different exercises. If you find that your fatigue level is going up, and your endurance is going down—the best answer may be that Power-*of*-10 should be an off-season activity for you.

5. How Long Before I See Real Results?

This depends on the quality of your workouts and your level of commitment to all 3 Pillars—Exercise, Nutrition, and Rest & Recovery. If you follow the basic prescriptions in Chapters 2, 3, and 4, you will start noticing real changes in the way you feel in 2 weeks. If you've got significant body fat to lose, you may see your average weight drop 2 to 3 pounds a week in the beginning, then you can expect to settle in at about 1 pound of weight loss per week—fat loss that's offset by muscle gain—until you reach your goal. Trust me, that's a lot of fat over time. Within 6 weeks of starting the program, you should really feel and see major results. Your clothes will be looser. Your body will feel leaner and tighter than ever. Your strength and energy levels will be noticeably improved, and people will be commenting on how good you look. From here, you can go to whatever level of fitness and body shape you want, just by continuing with the program.

6. What If I've Never Been to a Gym? Where Should I Start?

Everyone's had a first day at the gym when they looked at all the buff people and wondered how they'd ever fit in. Don't forget that every one of those folks had *their* first day, too. In any case, after you read the information in Part II, you'll be anything but a novice. You'll know more about the equipment and the proper execution of each exercise than the average gym veteran. To choose the right gym for you, just remember: every good gym knows it's a service business, first and foremost, and that means it must be a friendly, accommodating, and instructive place for everyone at any level. That attitude should come through to you loud and clear. Find a place that's convenient and ask for a tour. Check out the equipment on the floor and the dressing rooms. It should be clean and well maintained, period. Make sure they have all the major machines you'll be using in the Power-*of*-10 routines described in Part II. The staff should be knowledgeable and patient with all your questions. And they shouldn't be overly aggressive about sitting you down and signing you up on the spot if you're not ready. To me, that's a sign that they care more about collecting members than serving them. Finally, if possible, ask a member or two how they like the place. If you've got good vibes after your tour and your conversations with the staff, you've found your gym.

7. Can I Work Out at Home If a Gym's Not Available?

Yes, you can. I've included a series of routines and exercises for home workouts in Part II. You can take almost any home exercise, such as a push-up or sit-up, and turn it into a Power-*of*-10 exercise, simply by slowing down to the 10-second motion and attempting to reach failure. Likewise, you can perform any of the free weight exercises I describe in Chapter 6 at home with your own equipment. Machines at the gym just give you many, many more exercise options and they make it easier to progress because it's so simple to increase the weight as you get stronger. They're also safer because you can't pick up a machine and drop it.

8. What If I Want to Work Out Dressed as Mary Ann from Gilligan's Island?

So many people ask me this question, it's a matter of some debate among my staff. I actually think you'll have better results dressed as Ginger, as long as you remember to remove your high heels for the leg press.

9. How Important Is It to Use a Personal Trainer and Where Do I Find One?

I wrote this book so you wouldn't need to use a personal trainer to work out and get all the benefits of Power-*of*-10. That said, there's a reason why good coaches have a place in every athletic endeavor. They see things you don't see, they correct mistakes and help you make adjustments that only an objective pair of eyes can see. A good personal trainer is really just a good coach. If you have access to a trainer who is familiar with the slow-cadence principles of Power-*of*-10 training, the chances are your sessions will be worth the trainer's fee. All gyms have lists of trainers you can call. Trainers also advertise in local newspapers. The key is to find out whether they are knowledgeable about the Power-*of*-10 high-intensity, slow-cadence principles in general—or are willing to get knowledgeable by reading this book—so they can coach you effectively in the method you prefer. Just be forewarned that most trainers still come from the conventional school of weight lifting and will tend to talk you into what they're familiar with. That generally means 3 to 4 days a week at the gym plus aerobics and, in my opinion, a far greater risk of injury.

Q & A

10. Is Power-of-10 Safe for Older People?

I've taught Power-*of*-10 to clients of every age—from teenagers to eighty-year-olds. Several of my clients, in fact, are doctors in their sixties and seventies. Statistically and anecdotally, I know that there is no safer strength training method available today. Remember that Power-*of*-10 principles were first discovered in a study with older women who couldn't tolerate standard weight lifting motions, but were able to handle 10 second cadences with far fewer injuries and faster results. Just follow the rules of correct form; especially the good-breathing commandment. And I strongly recommend that you check first with your physician, especially if you have any prior medical condition, before undertaking any form of serious exercise.

11. Is It Safe for People with Heart Conditions?

If you have a preexisting heart condition, do not start any exercise program without consulting your doctor. When done properly, Power-*of*-10 is strenuous exercise, and any such exercise should be cleared first by your physician.

12. Is Power-of-10 Safe If You're Pregnant?

Again, check first with your doctor. However, it's commonly accepted today that sensible exercise can be very beneficial to the health of both pregnant mothers and their babies. Labor and delivery are extremely strenuous physical activities that women should get in shape for like any athlete, with proper muscular and metabolic conditioning. The irony is that most women let themselves become severely deconditioned during pregnancy, resulting in a greater chance of difficulties during labor—and afterward, a much longer period of recovery.

I've had several clients who were training with Power-*of*-10 when they got pregnant. They continued until the middle of their eighth month with very positive results. But I've always insisted that they be cleared by their doctor first.

13. What If I Feel Pain During My Workout?

There's muscle burn and then there's pain. Know the difference. Muscle burn is the discomfort in your muscles associated with muscle failure, the "good burn" that tells you the exercise is working. As I explained in Chapter 2, this burn says you've reached a crucial point in each set. You should push past it into muscle failure and sustain the push for at least 10 seconds as you become more advanced. There's also the normal muscle soreness you may encounter a day or two after your workout, especially at the beginning. That's okay too. *Almost all other pain is a potential harm signal*, and must be heeded. Sharp, stabbing pains in a muscle or in your joints can indicate a tear, a joint injury, or tendonitis, which will only get more inflamed, or worse, with continued use. This type of pain means you need to stop, rest the area in pain, and seek treatment if necessary. Unusual pains in the chest are obviously another major no-no. Quit your workout and see your doctor without delay. In general, a slight ache here or there is to be expected with any kind of exercise, especially the older we get. Just pay attention to what your body is telling you. If it's new, if it's sharp—"stop, look, and listen."

14. Can I Overdo the Burn?

It's really not possible to burn too much in your final rep. In fact, the safest rep in the set is your last one—the one where you're feeling the burn. At this point, you don't have enough strength left to generate the force that could cause an injury to your muscles or joints. The feeling of the burn is merely an indicator of fatigue and is not harmful in itself.

15. Can I Work Out When I Have a Cold or Am Sick?

If you don't have the energy to work out due to a cold or mild illness, your body's telling you it wants to rest. Let it. Be aware that the stress of any intense athletic exercise may temporarily lower your resistance, especially if you're already fighting something. So, if you have a cold coming on, don't feel guilty. Lie low and let it pass. As with all medical issues, when in doubt, ask your doctor.

16. As a Woman, I Want to Look Lean and Sculpted. Will Power-of-10 Make Me Bulk Up?

It's a myth that strength training makes women bulk up. Since lean muscle is more compact than fat, strength training will actually take off inches, making you smaller, rather than larger. Testosterone is the main factor that causes men to get bigger, bulkier muscles than women. Since women have a fraction of the testosterone men have, they needn't worry about adding bulk. It's possible that some women may perceive a larger muscle volume over time. However, this is most often due to increasing muscle mass without following Pillar 2, that is, without reducing the fat overlaying the muscles by following proper nutrition. Weight training plus proper nutrition is the fastest, most surefire way to achieve the lean, sculpted, and youthful look most of us want. Nearly all female celebrities who exercise work out with weights.

17. Should I Do More Reps at Lighter Weights If I Want to Avoid Bulking Up?

This is another myth. Working out with lighter weights simply means you'll expend more time without changing your results. The goal is to reach failure as efficiently as possible. As outlined in Chapter 2, we generally prescribe approximately 8 reps to failure when you're just starting out. Most experienced people do 4 to 6 reps. You can lower your rep count to as little as 3 as you become more advanced. The amount of weight you use is determined by your "Time Until Failure" (TUF) goal. For a 3-rep TUF, you'll naturally use a heavier weight than for an 8-rep TUF.

18. Is There a Best Time of the Day to Exercise?

This is completely a matter of preference. Some people love the 5:00 A.M. slot. Others aren't awake mentally or physically until midafternoon. Some love late-night workouts, while others become so wired working out late at night, they never get to sleep. It's entirely up to you.

19. Do I Really Need to Reach Muscle Failure?

Yes.

20. How Do I Really Know I'm Reaching Muscle Failure?

You'll no longer be able to move the weight in the positive or lifting direction. Your muscles will be quivering, your breathing will be rapid, and you should be experiencing a certain amount of burn.

21. When Will I Know It's Time to Switch from Twice-a-Week to Once-a-Week?

You don't ever have to switch if you don't want to, but most people do. It often happens all by itself. As you get more experienced, you'll probably find that it feels good to increase the weight and intensity. When you're reaching full muscle failure, your body will ask for more rest—generally 5 to 7 days between workouts—so you'll end up doing once-a-week by default. If you're a beginner and want to switch to once-a-week for convenience, I suggest you work out for at least 4 to 6 weeks before you attempt to switch, just to give yourself enough time and practice with the protocols. If you're doing 4 or 5 exercises in your twice-a-week workouts, you'll probably want to increase to 5 or 6 exercises, and add a little more weight to get a shorter, more intense TUF for your once-a-week program. Make the switch and see how it feels. Are you still making progress each week? Do you feel as energetic? After 5 or 6 days off, is your body ready for its next workout, or do you need a little more rest? Your body will give you the answers. Beyond that, it's really personal preference.

22. What Happens When I Travel or Go on Vacation?

What happens? The airline loses your luggage and Motel 66 puts you on a floor full of kids on spring break, that's what. Since you're not getting any sleep, and your gym clothes are on a flight to Alaska, I suggest you focus on the Pillars of Nutrition and Rest & Recovery, and forget working out till you get home. But if you really want to work out, find a local health club, pay the daily walk-in fee, and show all the civilians how we do it!

23. How Fast Will the Fat Come Off?

Metabolically, a person can lose a maximum of about 2 to 3 real pounds of fat a week. Any other weight loss will be "phantom" weight—water and fluids. In the beginning, depending on how much excess fat you have, and how carefully you adhere to the nutrition plan, the weight may come off at this relatively high rate. Later, most people level out at about 1 real pound of fat a week. That's a lot of fat over time. Again, remember that even though you're losing the fat, you'll be gaining muscle mass from exercise, so your losses on the scale may not reflect all the tightening and trimming that's happening to your body. You'll keep losing fat until your ratio of muscle to fat stabilizes at a natural, healthy equilibrium, which I promise you will be a higher state of fitness than you've ever experienced. At that point, you can adjust the program or maintain your level, based on your individual goals.

24. How Quickly Will I Notice Results?

You'll feel trimmer in the first week. You'll notice small changes, like your clothes getting looser, after 2 weeks. After 6 weeks of adherence to The 3 Pillars, people will be commenting about your appearance.

25. What About Taking Weight Loss Supplements?

The one supplement I take every day and that I recommend for everyone is a high-quality multivitamin and mineral combination. No matter how carefully we eat nowadays, a top-quality multivitamin and mineral supplement is the best insurance policy for optimal nutrition. Beyond vitamins, nearly every other supplement, particularly the weight loss enhancers, are highly controversial. They're either miracle substances or dangerous, depending on which expert you listen to. There are "fat-blocker" drugs, but these may also block the transport of vitamins and vital nutrients into your cells. There are also metabolic enhancers like ephedra. These are really just another form of the stimulant "speed" and, like speed, they make you nervous and jittery; and they can be outright dangerous if you have high blood pressure. Take any supplements at your own risk, especially over the long term. At the very least, study the literature available in print or on the internet. Consult your doctor about weight loss supplements, and be aware that the government doesn't regulate their manufacture, so always choose a company with a reputation for quality. My advice: eat 6 balanced meals and snacks a day, take your daily multivitamin, and work on your perfect Power-*of*-10 form at the gym.

26. I'm Already on a Nutritional Program That Works for Me. Do I Have to Switch?

If you're following a program of balanced nutrition that's not a diet but a long-term nutritional path, and if you are comfortably achieving the results you want, why rock the boat? Consider changing only if you're not reaching your strength, energy, and appearance goals.

27. What If I Don't Have Time to Eat 6 Times a Day?

Eating 6 times a day is an optimal goal. Sometimes time or other circumstances don't permit. Do your best At the very least, try to avoid going over 4 hours without eating so you don't activate the starvation response. Remember that the fewer meals you eat, the more critical it is to balance each one with protein, vegetables, grains, or legumes and fiber. And don't forget to drink your water.

28. Does It Help to Talk with a Nutritionist?

A good nutritionist is like any good coach. She can be a supporter, a motivator, and a mentor. Beware of any nutritionist who promises too miraculous or rapid results or who advocates a program too removed from the basics. No matter what anyone says, you can't live on a diet of grapefruit and water.

29. Should I Consult My Doctor?

Certainly talk to your doctor about nutrition if you have other questions, especially if you have a preexisting medical condition or allergies that might prevent you from eating certain foods.

30. Is There Such a Thing as Too Much Rest?

There's such a thing as too much of anything. If you rest for too many days between workouts—say, for 2 weeks—your muscles will pass the point of recovery and start to diminish in size and strength through lack of stimulation. Five to seven days between once-a-week workouts, and 3 to 4 days between twice-a-week workouts, seem to be the optimal rest periods for most people.

31. What If I've Tried Everything and Still Can't Sleep at Night?

Your doctor should be able to help. Ask him or her to recommend a good sleep therapist or sleep disorder clinic.

32. What About Sleep Aids or Medications?

Every sleep aid on the market is capable of becoming physically or psychologically habit forming. My advice is to avoid them. If you do try an occasional sleep aid and find yourself depending on it, you should let your doctor know immediately.

33. Is There Really a Sandman?

Yes, and you'll find that he visits you the night after each Power-*of*-10 workout. Then he goes home to New Jersey.

Don DiPaolo age 26

MUSICIAN

"I'm Not Just Stronger Now, I'm Healthier"

My entire life I was a skinny kid. I never really felt good about my body and had always wished I weighed more and was more muscle bound. So as soon as I was old enough, I got a membership at a gym and began every method and program under the sun. Weights, cardio, supersets, "pyramid sets," high reps light, low reps heavy—whatever there was, I tried it, 4 to 5 days every week. And still I never got anywhere! I was still too thin, without much muscle.

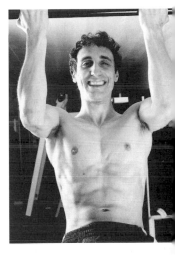

Then a year ago, a friend told me about Adam and Power-*of*-10. This wasn't just any friend, this guy was a martial arts expert who looked like my ideal—150 pounds of pure, ripped, muscular definition. He was doing Power-*of*-10 and claimed it took him just 20 minutes, once a week, and he was getting quicker, better results than with any other training. He was the perfect advertisement. A walking Power-*of*-10 billboard. So I went down that day to see Adam.

I loved it from day one. I felt totally present in my body; the workout made me feel the involvement of every muscle. I have a different feeling after my Power-*of*-10 workouts. A good intense feeling. My body feels happy after the workout.

It's a year later and I've reached my goals. I'm ripped, I'm so much stronger, and have had zero injuries. I feel really good about my body. However, it's not just the physical changes, I also feel healthier. I recommend Power *of* 10 to everyone.

Lori Jackson age 48

PERSONAL TRAINER

The Aerobics Instructor Who Gave Up on Aerobics . . .

I taught aerobics for 10 years. I hate to go on record saying this, but . . . I watched people who were so dedicated, they'd get up and exercise before work every morning, and for the most part I'd see the same bodies year after year. These people were killing themselves, and never seeing the changes they or I wanted to see. I finally had to admit that I wasn't helping these people the way I wanted to.

My clients started bringing me articles about slow-cadence strength training, and asking me what I knew. The claims were so fantastic, and the workout sounded so interesting, I decided to learn about it for my clients. I wanted to see if it was possible for a woman over 40 to actually improve the way she looked. We have all these hormone challenges—we normally gain weight as we age and lose muscle mass and bone density. So I'd tell my clients, if you're just holding the line that's good. I wanted to know if there was actually something that could make us look better. And the answer is yes.

I'm a perfect example. I've been with Adam for over a year now. I feel so much stronger. I've got energy to burn these days that I didn't have when I started. And as far as I look . . . the summer that I turned 47, right *before* I started Power-*of*-10, I got out all my summer stuff, my bikini, my sundresses—I sighed in distress and threw them all away! On my forty-eighth birthday—the summer *after* I found Power-*of*-10, I bought three bikinis. I wore them and felt really comfortable. That's a pretty big deal!

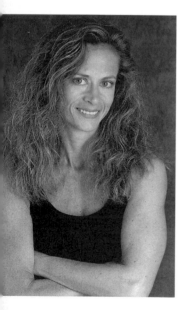

My legs have a new shape. My butt is higher; it's actually lifted up. I have more definition in my hamstrings and especially my quads. Last year I didn't even want to wear shorts, and this year I felt really comfortable with short-shorts. After pregnancy, my arms were looking a little flabby and that's improved, too.

What's most surprising—I'm a certified aerobics instructor and cardiovascular activity is the be-all and end-all in that type of training. But when Adam said you never have to do that again, I just took a complete leap of faith. I have these results, and *I have not done a stitch of cardiovascular activity in over a year*. I still do yoga once a week, but that's it.

I also haven't had any strains or injury since I started, and a chronic problem with neck pain has completely gone away. Power-*of*-10 always challenges me. I find that really good emotionally. And the fact that you can get it done in so little time each week is amazing. Today I train all my clients using Power-*of*-10. I wouldn't do it any other way.

POWER-of-10

PART II
THE POWER-OF-
10 STEP-BY-STEP
WORKOUT

Right now I'm imagining that you're standing in my studio, waiting for your very first workout. You're a little nervous. I'm a little relieved you're not the one who wanted to come dressed as Mary Ann from *Gilligan's Island*. As I open the gym door, I'm smiling because I can picture all the exciting changes that are about to happen . . .

IN THE GYM AND READY TO START

THE 5-MINUTE PRELAUNCH COUNTDOWN

Here's the 5 minute talk I give every new client as we walk around the workout room, getting ready for our first session. It's a basic equipment tour so you understand the correct body positions and operation of the machines at any gym, plus last-minute instructions, reminders, and hints that will help you start right from your first rep. In Chapter 6, you'll find complete illustrations of all my favorite routines, with each individual exercise shown in step-by-step form.

START WITH A CHART

The first thing you'll see me do is pull out a single blank form like the one on the following page.

	EXERCISE	DATE:					
	EXERCISE	SEAT ADJ.	WT / TUF	WT / TUF	WT / TUF	WT / TUF	WT / TUF
1							
2							
3							
4							
5							
6							
7							
8							
9							
10							
11							
12							

Just make copies of the blank form (or download it from my website, www.power-of-10.com) and fill it in as I've shown below. Believe me, this isn't busywork. The chart will save you time and give you a sense of being in control of your fitness program from day one. It provides the essential reference point from which to measure progress; it frees your mind to focus 100 percent on the exercise, instead of wondering if this is the machine that you set at 80 pounds at height 5, or 50 pounds at height 8. Remembering the adjustment settings on each machine is crucial. Changing the seat position from workout to workout, for example, will effect the amount of force you need to exert, giving you a false reading of your progress.

			A	B	A	B		
	EXERCISE	SEAT ADJ.	DATE: 9/9 WT / TUF	9/14 WT / TUF	9/19 WT / TUF	9/25 WT / TUF	WT / TUF	WT / TUF
1	LEG PRESS	#7	400 / 6 — 1 / 2:05		410 / 6 — 1 / 2:03			
2	LAT PULLDOWN	#6	50 / 7 — 2 / 2:30		55 / 6 — 2 / 2:00			
3	CHEST PRESS		100 / 6 — 3 / 1:50		100 / 6 — 3 / 2:00			
4	BICEPS CURL		50 / 4 — 4 / 1:20		45 / 5 — 4 / 1:32			
5	ABDOMINAL CRUNCH		BODY WT / 6 — 5		BODY WT / 6 — 5 / 1:40			
6	HAMSTRING CURL			120 / 3 — 1 / 1.00		100 / 4 — 1 / 1:20		
7	LEG EXTENSION			130 / 6 — 2 / 2:10		140 / 5 — 2 / 2:01		
8	COMPOUND ROW			200 / 7 — 3 / 2:30		210 / 6 — 3 / 2:15		
9	LATERAL RAISE			40 / 3 — 4 / 1:55		30 / 5 — 4 / 1:40		
10	BACK EXTENSION			BODY WEIGHT — 5 / 1:20		BODY WEIGHT — 5 / 1:35		
11								
12								

A TYPICAL PROGRESS CHART

KEY: For example, for the leg press, the seat position is set at #7; the weight used is 400 pounds; the number of reps is 6; the order in which the exercise is performed is 1st; and the time until failure is 2:05.

MACHINE BASICS

When you look into a room full of exercise machines for the first time, they may seem like a bunch of big, complicated contraptions. But taken one at a time, today's machines are very simple, designed to be adjusted in seconds. All machines require you to set the weight, and to adjust one or two moving parts to match the size and motion of your body. Every gym has an attendant on duty who will show you how to set any machine in a few seconds. Once the machine is ready, don't forget to note the settings on your chart so you won't have to guess next time. Beyond that, there are really just two basic kinds of machines you have to know about.

Rotary Machines for "Simple Exercises"

Rotary machines are designed to match the motion of one specific body part as it rotates around one specific "axis" joint. In a biceps curl, for example, your elbow is the axis joint, and the forearm is the rotating body part or lever arm. The machine has an axis joint and a steel lever arm, too. All rotary machines are designed to easily adjust the seat height, length of lever arm, and sometimes range of motion, so they line up with the axis of rotation of your body. Proper adjustment not only makes the machine most efficient, it also prevents injury by balancing the stress on joints and muscles.

Exercises that isolate and work the muscles around one joint at a time, like the biceps curl or the leg extension, are called "simple exercises." Simple exercises are generally performed on rotary machines.

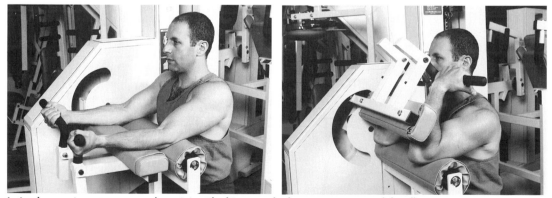

A simple exercise rotates around one joint. The biceps curl, above, rotates around the elbow.

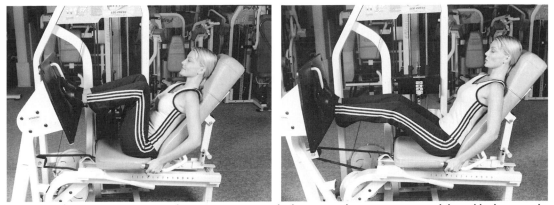

A compound exercise rotates around two or more joints. The leg press, above, rotates around the ankle, knee, and hips.

Compound Motion Machines for "Compound Exercises"

In contrast to rotary machines, any equipment that involves two or more joints at a time is called a "compound motion machine" and is used to perform "compound exercises." The leg press is a good example of a compound exercise. As you push the legs forward against the platform, you move your ankle joints and your knee and hip joints. In the process, you involve many more muscle groups than you would in a simple motion exercise, causing deeper levels of fatigue. Because so many axis joints and motions are involved, most compound machines can't be lined up with each of your joints like rotary machines can, so even though they're called "compound," they often have fewer adjustments.

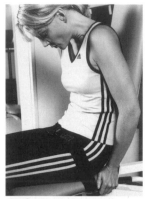

"Body C" position

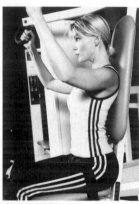

"Ten-Hut!" position

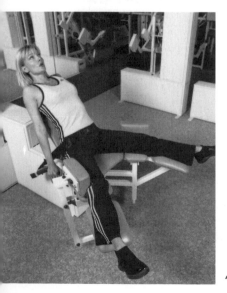

"2-second squeeze" technique

SPECIAL BODY POSTURES AND TECHNIQUES TO BOOST RESULTS

There are some exercises where simply sitting a certain way, or pausing at a certain time, makes a big enough difference for me to include it in the exercise description. These are refinements that set you up for perfect form. So, when I describe an exercise, if you see "Special Posture: *'Body C,'* or *'Ten-Hut!'* or the *'2-Second Squeeze,'*" the following is what I mean. And don't worry, whenever an exercise calls for it, I'll state it clearly.

1. **THE "BODY C":** Sit with your hips tilted upward, and your shoulders rolled forward, the middle of your back against the seat pad, like you're forming the letter C with your body.

2. **THE "TEN-HUT!":** Sit or stand with your chest up, and your shoulders back and down during the exercise, just like a soldier who snaps to attention when the sergeant says, *"Ten-Hut!"*

3. **THE "2-SECOND SQUEEZE" TECHNIQUE:** At the very top of the first rep, pause and hold for a 2-second contraction of your muscles before you reverse direction and let the weight down. It's a results-boosting technique that can be used with many of the simple, rotary machine exercises like the biceps curl or lateral raise. All you do is pause for a moment at the top of your circle of power and intensify your muscle contraction, then begin the negative rep that takes you back down. Holding the squeeze in rotary exercises like these is not like cheating or locking out, because your muscles have to work full force to hold the squeeze—they're not resting or "unloading" in any way.

FINAL MACHINE HINTS

- **USE YOUR SEAT BELT!** Always buckle the seat belts that are included with certain machines, and buckle them tightly. Seat belts lock you down so that less motion is wasted, and the main focus of effort is on the target muscles where you want it. Seat belts also help prevent injury.

- **"PINNING THE STACK."** Pinning the weight stack is an optional but effective way to limit a machine's range of motion, if that range goes beyond what's safe for your body. By pinning the weight stack, you can stop some machines from causing over-stretch, and ensure that you'll always perform each rep with the same range of motion. As the illustration shows, simply remove the selector pin, push the machine movement arms up a few pin slots to where you want the motion to start and stop, and replace the pin. Pinning the stack doesn't change the amount of weight you're lifting, it just shortens the distance the weight stack can travel. Pinning the stack isn't a requirement, it's a trick you can use to adjust some machines more perfectly to your body.

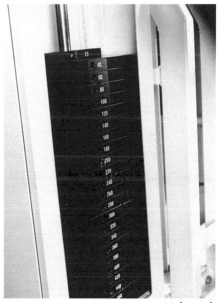

Weight stack

- **MACHINE CHEATING POINTS.** Every machine has a list of what I call "cheating points"—the most common ways people tend to break form on that particular machine. I'll list them when we get to each specific exercise.

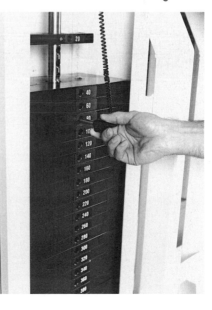

Pinned weight stack

THE ROUTINES AND THE EXERCISES

Since we exercise the full body in a Power-*of*-10 workout, we have to choose a mix of exercises that covers all the body parts in each session. We need to balance the number of compound and simple motion exercises so we don't burn ourselves out too quickly or overtrain. We need to perform the exercises in the right order: large muscle groups first, then smaller, so we warm up efficiently and optimize our energy for the whole session. And we need to vary our exercises from time to time, to stimulate a wider variety of muscle fibers and simply prevent boredom.

Structuring routines is so important, the last thing you should do is try to guess (or stress) at this point. In the next chapter, I illustrate 12 of my favorites, organized into twice-a-week routines, once-a-week routines, and home-and-travel routines. Exercise by exercise, I'll indicate the muscle group trained, whether it's compound or simple; and I'll show the correct order so you can start with total confidence. For quick reference, next to each of the listed exercises you'll find the page where that exercise is shown in complete detail. As you get more experienced, you'll be able to create your own routines from the individual exercise section, or substitute similar exercises from one routine into another. But even if you stick with my 12 favorite routines forever, you'll have enough variety for a whole lifetime of Power-*of*-10 exercise.

MAGIC WORDS FOR EVERY EXERCISE YOU DO

At this point I'm buckling you into the first machine, and these are my final words of wisdom. Believe me, no one follows them all at first. I could talk till I'm blue in the face, and you're still going to speed up when the burn sets in, or hold your breath when you begin the push at the start of a rep—because everybody does at first. But that's what coaches are for. Even pro athletes have coaches who whisper something in their ear before they run into the game for the thousandth time. These are the special words I'd say to you:

- **THE MOST IMPORTANT REP IS THE ONE YOU'RE ON.** The first rep is as important as the last. Just focus on your most perfect form and speed at each moment, and true muscle failure will happen in the time and manner it's supposed to.

- **AIM FOR 10 SECONDS UP AND 10 SECONDS DOWN, BUT . . .** In the beginning, if you have trouble holding your cadence that long, or if an occasional machine has sticky points that throw you off a little, don't worry. Eight seconds or twelve seconds is acceptable—as long as you reach muscle failure at the end of your set.

- **NEVER "BLAST OUT OF THE BOX" WHEN YOU BEGIN EACH REP.** Start slowly, gradually; squeeze the weight forward.

- **DON'T HOLD YOUR BREATH WHEN YOU START EACH REP, OR WHEN YOU'RE TRYING TO SQUEEZE OUT YOUR LAST FEW SECONDS.** Nothing is more important than full, continuous breathing through every moment of every exercise.

- **TRY MOUTHING THE WORD "HA-A" AS YOU BREATHE.** It helps keep you from tightening up your face, gritting your teeth, or generally tensing your body as you go.

- **DON'T SPEED UP OR CHANGE YOUR FORM TO FINISH YOUR LAST REP.** The number of reps DOES NOT MATTER. We only care about the correct form that takes us to muscle failure.

- **DON'T SQUIRM AROUND OR CHANGE YOUR BODY POSTURE TO FINISH YOUR LAST REP.** Keep stable, calm, and steady.

- **WHEN YOU NO LONGER CAN MOVE THE WEIGHT, KEEP PUSHING FOR 10 MORE SECONDS.**

- **IF THE BURN STARTS AFTER 2 OR 3 REPS, DON'T THINK YOU'RE WEAK.** You're firing deeper layers of muscle fiber than ever before, and you're experiencing how efficient Power-*of*-10 really is!

- **DON'T EXPECT TO BE STRONG OR PERFECT ON DAY ONE.** No one is. You will be soon.

- **ENOUGH REMEMBERING. HERE ARE TWO THINGS YOU CAN FORGET!** *You don't have to warm up or stretch before or after the workout if you don't want to!* You'll recall from Part One that the warm-up and stretching are *built-into* Power-*of*-10 because of the slow speed and complete range of motion. Just pick a routine, grab a machine, and start right in. You certainly can stretch or warm up if you like—but do it in moderation. It's optional.

In the beginning, you'll be constantly correcting yourself, using your own mental checklist as you ask: "Am I going too fast?" "Am I pushing smoothly out of the box?" "Am I keeping my face relaxed?" "Am I breathing throughout?" "Am I staying focused on each and every rep?" "Am I getting to failure?" But with a little time and experience, the form becomes natural, and that zen-like focus I've talked about will arrive all on its own.

It's workout time!

Lloyd Morrisett age 71

FOUNDER OF SESAME WORKSHOP, WHICH CREATED *SESAME STREET*

At 71, He Needed Muscle Mass, Not Pain, Injury, or a Hectic Routine . . .

In the last 2 years I realized I needed to do strength training. I was losing muscle as I was getting older. But I didn't want to take time from all my other activities. Then a friend of mine told me about a *Newsweek* article and getting all your training once a week, so I called Adam's studio and made a date.

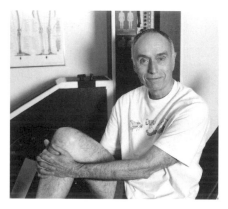

I started with Power-*of*-10 and liked it immediately. I'm clearly stronger than when I began, there's no doubt about that. Anywhere between 25 and 40 percent stronger, depending on the exercise. For the first several months, for 1 to 3 days after the session, I felt more like resting than exercising. Now I'm also swimming 3 to 5 times a week. I'm stronger in the arm motion of the crawl, and also the backstroke. I've certainly noticed that in doing things like going up long flights of stairs I'm not tired at the end, whereas I might have been before.

When I do my Power-*of*-10 workouts, I really like the feeling of having done all that you could possibly do. I also enjoy the emphasis on safety. It's highly important for older people. You do this in such a way that you don't have any sudden stresses on your body, and that saves lots of injuries, as Adam points out.

I recommend the workout to everybody.

Lisa Jubilee age 29

NUTRITIONIST

After 8 Years Trying Other Methods, Power-of-10 Got Her to Her Goal . . .

For 8 years I trained the traditional gym way. Three sets of 10, 4 or 5 days a week. It used to drive me crazy making the time because I'm so busy, and I'm a nutritionist so I'm expected to look good—but I could never seem to lose that last 5 pounds no matter what I did. I heard about Adam from one of his trainers I met at a club. He told me I could get better results working out once or twice a week for less than half an hour! It definitely sounded too good to be true, but he looked great and I trusted him, so I decided to try something different.

Adam recommended that I start with twice-a-week to get adjusted. In 4 weeks I was noticing these changes. I was getting leaner in the legs and in the waist, and my abs were getting this new definition. Within a few more weeks, I started shedding body fat, even though my hunger was increasing and I was eating more! It seemed miraculous but it was happening. I switched to one workout per week after about the sixth week.

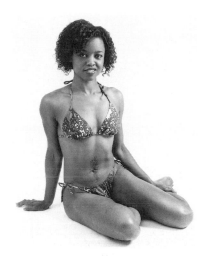

Today I do only 6 exercises in 1 workout each week and I've never been in better personal shape. My whole routine is done in about 15 minutes. I'd never believe it if it hadn't happened to me. My tennis game is better. My energy and endurance are really high. I'm totally happy with my body for the first time in my life. I love that Power-of-10 produces more results in less time. The choice is between 15 really focused minutes once a week, or 5 days a week in the gym. I'll never do anything else and I recommend it to every single one of my clients.

TWICE-A-WEEK ROUTINES—THE *BEST* WAY TO START

I *strongly* recommend that you start with twice-a-week routines, whether you're an experienced weight trainer or a complete beginner. Twice-a-week gets you comfortable more quickly with

6

ROUTINES AND EXERCISES

the form and cadence of Power-*of*-10. And it doesn't require the focus or efficiency that once-a-week does right off the bat. Remember that you can stay with twice-a-week forever, or move to once-a-week in a month or so, whenever it feels right. It's entirely your preference.

In all the routines that follow, we mix compound and simple exercises, work the entire body, and progress from larger to smaller muscle groups. *That's why it's important to perform the exercises in the specific order I've listed.*

Picking the Right Weight and Number of Starting Reps

For your convenience, I'll recap some of the points I made in Chapter 2 about starting weights and reps. If you have time, it wouldn't hurt to go back and do a quick review of that chapter as you get into the actual physical part of the program.

In the beginning—even if you're already in shape—I want you to pick a lighter weight where you reach muscle failure by about the eighth rep. Since each full rep lasts 20 seconds, that means you'll fail in about 2 minutes and 40 seconds (160 seconds). It takes 3 to 4 workouts of trial and error on the different machines before you settle on the perfect weight. But I promise—after a few workouts, *the right weight will find you!* The first time, pick any reasonable looking weight and start your set. You may blow right past 8 reps to 10 or more. Or you might konk out at 5. Next workout, add a few pounds if the weight's too light, or remove a few if it's too heavy, it's as simple as that. Within a few workouts, you'll zero in on that weight that allows you 8 reps before muscle failure. From there, we start measuring regular progress.

Stick with the 8-rep count for a while until you're really feeling comfortable and confident with the program. When you get stronger and more experienced, 6, 5, 4, or even 3 reps may be preferable in terms of time and effectiveness. What matters most is that you keep form, motion, and speed—and that you take yourself to muscle failure.

Choosing the Routines

Mix and match any way you like. You can stick with one routine forever, or change week to week for variety. With each routine, the exercises are meant to be done in order, but the routines themselves are interchangeable.

THE ROUTINES

Twice-a-Week Routine 1

- Perform exercises in order.

- Beginners—set weight to reach muscle failure in about 8 reps.

- Go from exercise to exercise with minimum delay.

SESSION 1

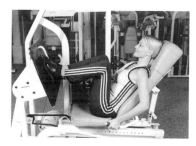

START. LEG PRESS

PAGE 112

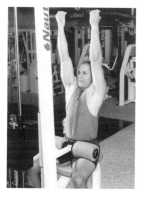

2. LAT PULLDOWN

PAGE 152

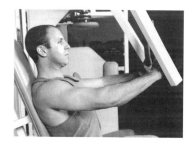

3. CHEST PRESS

PAGE 144

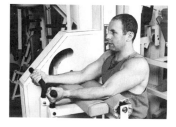

4. BICEPS CURL

PAGE 180

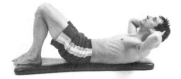

5. AB CRUNCH

PAGE 164

REST 3–5 DAYS

- Record in your chart.

- When an exercise lists a variety, like ab crunches or compound rows, choose whichever you like.

SESSION 2

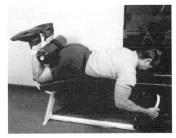

START. HAMSTRING CURL

PAGE 114

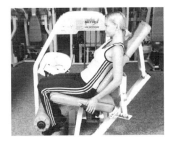

2. LEG EXTENSION

PAGE 116

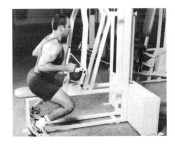

3. COMPOUND ROW

PAGE 154

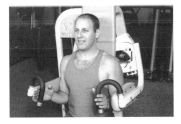

4. LATERAL RAISE

PAGE 138

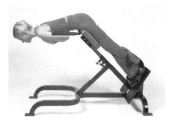

5. BACK EXTENSION, ROMAN CHAIR

PAGE 174

Twice-a-Week Routine 2

- Perform exercises in order.

- Beginners—set weight to reach muscle failure in about 8 reps.

- Go from exercise to exercise with minimum delay.

SESSION 1

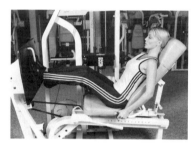

START. LEG PRESS

PAGE 112

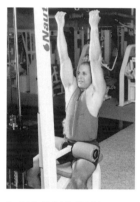

2. LAT PULLDOWN

PAGE 152

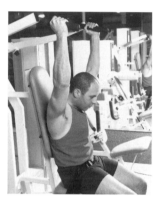

3. SHOULDER PRESS

PAGE 134

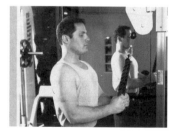

4. TRICEPS EXTENSION

PAGE 186

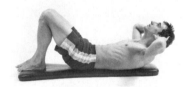

5. AB CRUNCH

PAGE 164

> **REST 3–5 DAYS**

- Record in your chart.
- When an exercise lists a variety, like ab crunches or compound rows, choose whichever you like.

SESSION 2

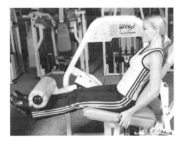

START. LEG EXTENSION

PAGE 116

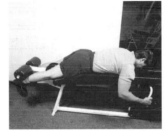

2. HAMSTRING CURL

PAGE 114

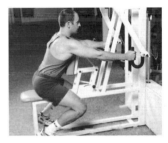

3. COMPOUND ROW

PAGE 154

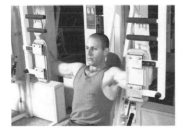

4. CHEST FLYE

PAGE 146

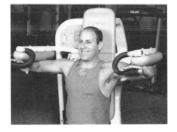

5. LATERAL RAISE

PAGE 138

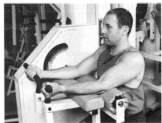

6. BICEPS CURL

PAGE 180

Twice-a-Week Routine 3

- Perform exercises in order.

- Beginners—set weight to reach muscle failure in about 8 reps.

- Go from exercise to exercise with minimum delay.

SESSION 1

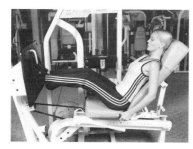

START. LEG PRESS

PAGE 112

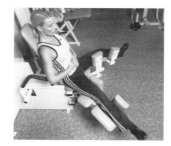

2. HIP ADDUCTION

PAGE 126

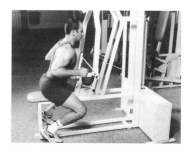

3. COMPOUND ROW

PAGE 154

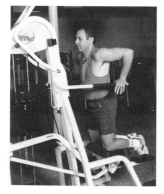

4. DIP WITH MACHINE

PAGE 136

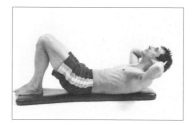

5. AB CRUNCH

PAGE 164

> REST 3–5 DAYS

- Record in your chart.
- When an exercise lists a variety, like ab crunches or compound rows, choose whichever you like.

SESSION 2

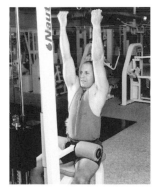

START. CALF RAISE

PAGE 118

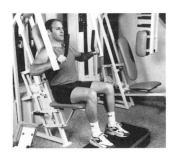

2. LEG EXTENSION

PAGE 116

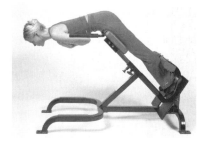

3. HIP ABDUCTION

PAGE 128

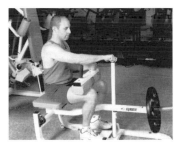

4. LAT PULLDOWN

PAGE 152

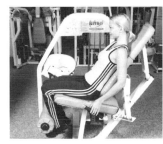

5. CHEST PRESS

PAGE 144

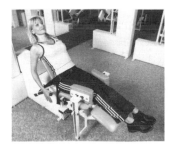

6. BACK EXTENSION, ROMAN CHAIR

PAGE 174

Twice-a-Week Routine 4 (Split Routine)

Since there's an exception to every rule—in this case, the rule that we exercise the whole body in every workout—I've included this split routine for variety. In split routines, we exercise only the upper body in one session, the lower body in the next session. It still adds up to the whole body being exercised in 1 week. Split routines are a little more demanding, so beginners should wait to try them until they've had more practice.

SESSION 1

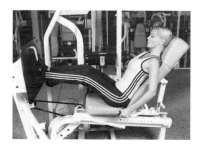

START. LEG PRESS
PAGE 112

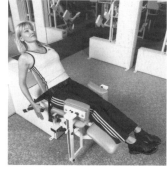

2. HIP ABDUCTION
PAGE 128

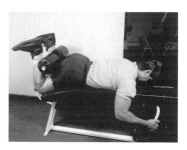

3. HAMSTRING CURL
PAGE 114

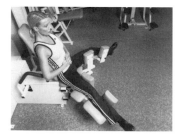

4. HIP ADDUCTION
PAGE 126

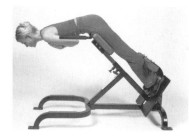

5. BACK EXTENSION, ROMAN CHAIR
PAGE 174

REST 3–5 DAYS

- Perform exercises in order.

- Beginners—set weight to reach muscle failure in about 8 reps.

- Go from exercise to exercise with minimum delay.

- Record in your chart.

- When an exercise lists a variety, like ab crunches or compound rows, choose whichever you like.

SESSION 2

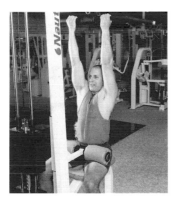

START. LAT PULLDOWN

PAGE 152

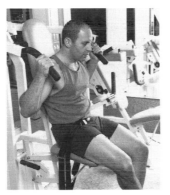

2. SHOULDER PRESS

PAGE 134

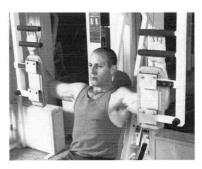

3. CHEST FLYE

PAGE 146

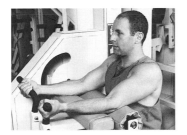

4. BICEPS CURL

PAGE 180

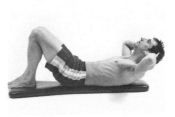

5. AB CRUNCH

PAGE 164

ONCE-A-WEEK ROUTINES

When to Switch to Once-a-Week

As I've said, there's no right or wrong time to switch, and some people may decide they prefer twice-a-week and stick with it permanently. My main advice is to give yourself at least 3 or 4 weeks of trial and adjustment before you make the switch. For once-a-week to be most effective, your form and your ability to reach muscle failure are more important because you're giving yourself just one chance to fire all your muscle fibers and "flip all your switches." That usually requires some practice.

Many of my twice-a-week clients evolve to once a week simply by default. They get so efficient, achieving such excellent muscle fatigue and muscle failure, their bodies no longer recover in 3 to 4 days. They need 5 to 7 days of rest. Voilà! They're exercising once a week automatically.

Routines That Emphasize Different Body Parts

All the routines exercise the whole body, but I've also included some that emphasize certain areas over others for those who want to concentrate more on a particular group of muscles. Again, as you get more advanced, you can create your own routines, taking anything you want from the individual exercises listed in the next section.

Once-a-Week Routine 1

- Perform exercises in order.

- Beginners set weight to reach muscle failure in about 8 reps—twice-a-week routines recommended to start.

- Go from exercise to exercise with minimum delay.

- Record in your chart.

- When an exercise lists a variety, like ab crunches or compound rows, choose whichever you like.

- Rest 5 to 7 days.

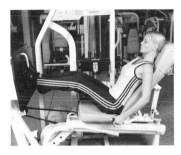

START. LEG PRESS

PAGE 112

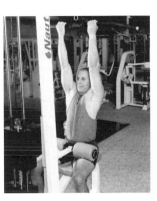

2. LAT PULLDOWN

PAGE 152

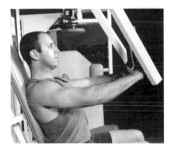

3. CHEST PRESS

PAGE 144

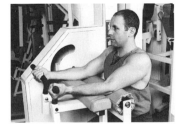

4. BICEPS CURL

PAGE 180

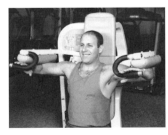

5. LATERAL RAISE

PAGE 138

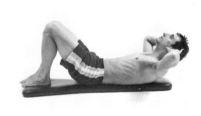

6. AB CRUNCH

PAGE 164

Once-a-Week Routine 2

- Perform exercises in order.
- Beginners set weight to reach muscle failure in about 8 reps—twice-a-week routines recommended to start.
- Go from exercise to exercise with minimum delay.
- Record in your chart.
- When an exercise lists a variety, like ab crunches or compound rows, choose whichever you like.
- Rest 5 to 7 days.

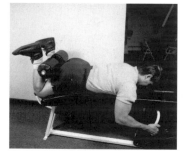

START. HAMSTRING CURL

PAGE 114

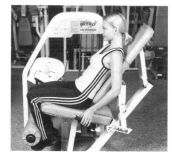

2. LEG EXTENSION

PAGE 116

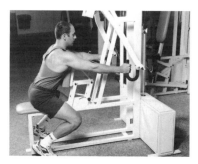

3. COMPOUND ROW

PAGE 154

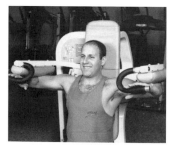

4. LATERAL RAISE

PAGE 138

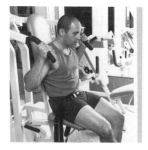

5. SHOULDER PRESS

PAGE 134

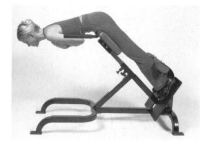

6. BACK EXTENSION, ROMAN CHAIR

PAGE 174

Once-a-Week Routine 3

- Perform exercises in order.

- Beginners—set weight to reach muscle failure in about 8 reps—twice-a-week routines recommended to start.

- Go from exercise to exercise with minimum delay.

- Record in your chart.

- When an exercise lists a variety, like ab crunches or compound rows, choose whichever you like.

- Rest 5 to 7 days.

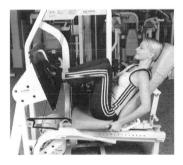

START. LEG PRESS

PAGE 112

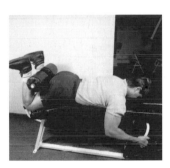

2. HAMSTRING CURL

PAGE 114

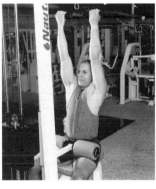

3. LAT PULLDOWN

PAGE 152

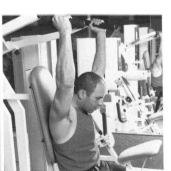

4. SHOULDER PRESS

PAGE 134

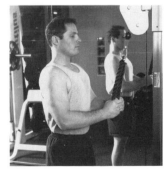

5. TRICEPS EXTENSION

PAGE 186

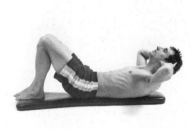

6. AB CRUNCH

PAGE 164

Once-a-Week Routine 4 (Chest and Shoulders Emphasis)

- Perform exercises in order.

- Beginners—set weight to reach muscle failure in about 8 reps—twice-a-week routines recommended to start.

- Go from exercise to exercise with minimum delay.

- Record in your chart.

- When an exercise lists a variety, like ab crunches or compound rows, choose whichever you like.

- Rest 5 to 7 days.

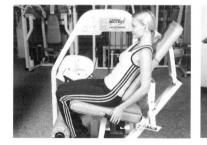

START. LEG EXTENSION

PAGE 116

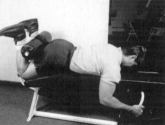

2. HAMSTRING CURL

PAGE 114

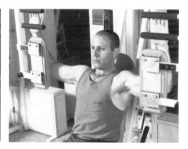

3. CHEST FLYE

PAGE 146

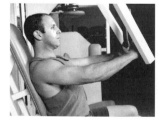

4. CHEST PRESS

PAGE 144

5. LATERAL RAISE

PAGE 138

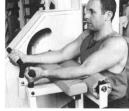

6. BICEPS CURL

PAGE 180

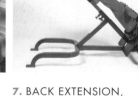

7. BACK EXTENSION, ROMAN CHAIR

PAGE 174

Once-a-Week Routine 5 (Hips and Buttocks Emphasis)

- Perform exercises in order.

- Beginners—set weight to reach muscle failure in about 8 reps—twice-a-week routines recommended to start.

- Go from exercise to exercise with minimum delay.

- Record in your chart.

- When an exercise lists a variety, like ab crunches or compound rows, choose whichever you like.

- Rest 5 to 7 days.

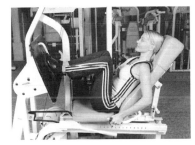

START. LEG PRESS

PAGE 112

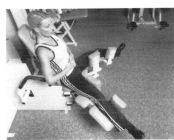

2. HIP ADDUCTION

PAGE 126

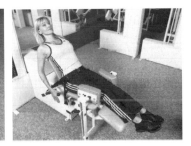

3. HIP ABDUCTION

PAGE 128

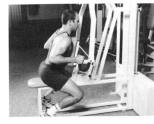

4. COMPOUND ROW

PAGE 154

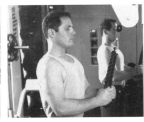

5. TRICEPS EXTENSION

PAGE 186

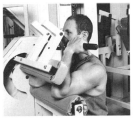

6. BICEPS CURL

PAGE 180

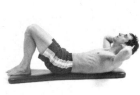

7. AB CRUNCH

PAGE 164

Once-a-Week Routine 6 (Legs Emphasis)

- Perform exercises in order.

- Beginners—set weight to reach muscle failure in about 8 reps—twice-a-week routines recommended to start.

- Go from exercise to exercise with minimum delay.

- Record in your chart.

- When an exercise lists a variety, like ab crunches or compound rows, choose whichever you like.

- Rest 5 to 7 days.

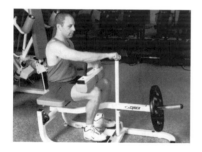

START. CALF RAISE

PAGE 118

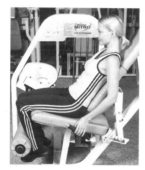

2. LEG EXTENSION

PAGE 116

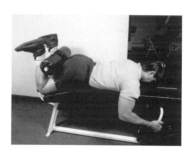

3. HAMSTRING CURL

PAGE 114

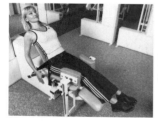

4. HIP ABDUCTION

PAGE 128

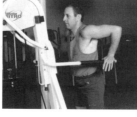

5. DIP WITH MACHINE

PAGE 136

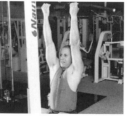

6. LAT PULLDOWN

PAGE 152

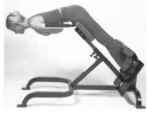

7. BACK EXTENSION, ROMAN CHAIR

PAGE 174

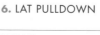

HOME AND TRAVEL ROUTINES

Home and travel routines are designed to use floors, walls, benches, chairs, doorways—and simple inexpensive exercise equipment like dumbbells, in some cases—so you can have a good workout when you can't go to your regular gym. Not that you *have* to go to the gym—these are all real, legitimate exercises that you can use to great effect. But the gym gives you so much more variety and such safe, high-quality equipment, just about everyone who takes up Power-*of*-10 eventually decides a good local gym is what they want long term. Home and travel routines can be performed either once or twice a week, based on your schedule, your preference, and the intensity you put into your workouts.

An Important Word of Caution on Free Weights

Many of the home exercises require the use of simple free weight barbells or dumbbells, which are relatively cheap and can be found at any sporting goods store. But please take care. Unlike machines, free weights carry an inherent extra risk: you could drop them on some part of you, especially when you reach muscle failure. For that reason, I only recommend specific free weight exercises where if the weight is dropped, it's not likely to land on your body. For example, I don't recommend that you do chest presses or shoulder presses in which you hold the barbell over your head. You can also cause serious muscle pulls by simply picking free weights up in an unbalanced or awkward manner. Never jerk them off the floor or reach for them from a careless stance. In the end, safety is up to you. Use common sense and you'll avoid injuries.

Simple Equipment for Home Workouts

You can give yourself an excellent Power-*of*-10 home workout with the following simple and relatively inexpensive equipment.

A padded "flat bench"

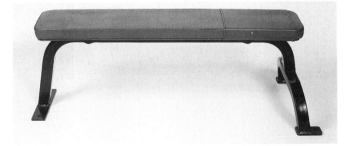

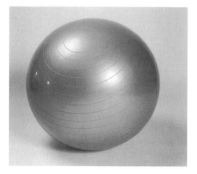

A large-diameter, air-filled "Workout Ball"

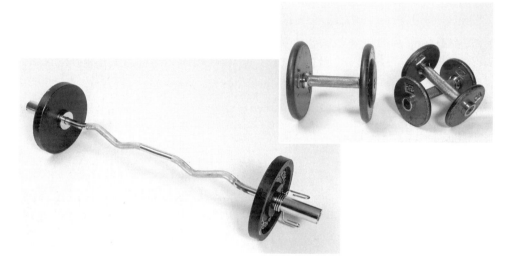

A barbell, preferably with the EZ Curl zigzag shape, and weight plates and/or a basic dumbbell set

- Perform exercises in order.

- Exercise until you reach muscle failure.

- Go from exercise to exercise with minimum delay.

- Record in your chart.

- When an exercise lists a variety, like ab crunches or biceps curls, choose whichever you like.

- Rest as needed, 3 to 7 days.

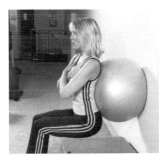

START. WALL SQUAT WITH BALL

PAGE 122

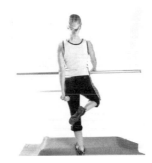

2. ONE-LEGGED CALF RAISE WITH FREE WEIGHTS

PAGE 120

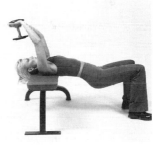

3. FLAT BENCH PULLOVER WITH FREE WEIGHTS

PAGE 160

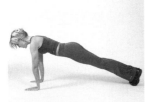

4. PUSH-UP

PAGE 148

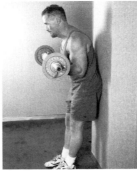

5. BICEPS CURL WITH FREE WEIGHTS

PAGE 182

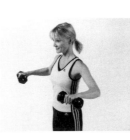

6. LATERAL RAISE WITH FREE WEIGHTS

PAGE 140

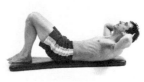

7. AB CRUNCH

PAGE 164

Home Routine 2

- Perform exercises in order.

- Exercise until you reach muscle failure.

- Go from exercise to exercise with minimum delay.

- Record in your chart.

- When an exercise lists a variety, like ab crunches or biceps curls, choose whichever you like.

- Rest as needed, 3 to 7 days.

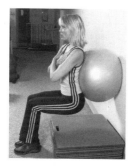

START. WALL SQUAT WITH BALL

PAGE 122

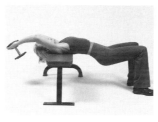

2. FLAT BENCH PULLOVER WITH FREE WEIGHTS

PAGE 160

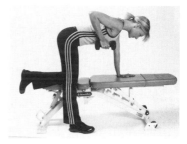

3. ONE-ARMED ROW WITH FREE WEIGHTS

PAGE 158

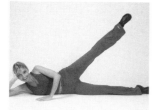

4. FLOOR ABDUCTION

PAGE 130

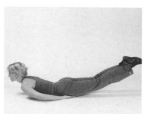
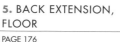

5. BACK EXTENSION, FLOOR

PAGE 176

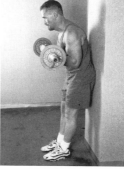
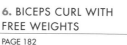

6. BICEPS CURL WITH FREE WEIGHTS

PAGE 182

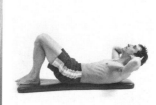

7. AB CRUNCH

PAGE 164

Travel Routine

This routine is for those of you who travel and happen to be in a hotel room with nothing but the floor and the wall to work with. While the routine is perfectly effective, keep in mind that you also have the option to walk into the local fitness center, or to use the hotel gym. Most are generally much improved from what they used to be.

- **Perform exercises in order.**

- **Exercise until you reach muscle failure.**

- **Go from exercise to exercise with minimum delay.**

- **Record in your chart.**

- **When an exercise lists a variety, like ab crunches or biceps curls, choose whichever you like.**

- **Rest as needed, 3 to 7 days.**

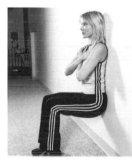

START. WALL SQUAT, STATIC HOLD

PAGE 124

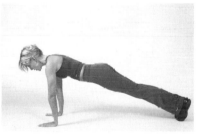

2. PUSH-UP

PAGE 148

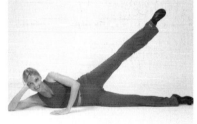

3. FLOOR ABDUCTION

PAGE 130

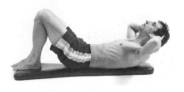

4. AB CRUNCH

PAGE 164

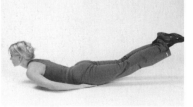

5. BACK EXTENSION, FLOOR

PAGE 176

THE EXERCISES

The exercises that follow are organized by major body groups: legs and hips, shoulders and neck, chest, back, core, and arms. Each exercise is also listed as either compound, involving multiple joints and muscles, or simple, involving the muscles around a single joint. Once you are more experienced, you can substitute any corresponding exercise into any of the routines, or create your own routines, following mix and match patterns similar to those I've outlined in the "Routines" section.

REMINDER ABOUT SPECIAL POSTURES

I'm going to be asking for the *"Body C,"* the *"Ten-Hut!"* or the *"2-second squeeze"* in many of the upcoming rotary machine exercises. Remember, the Body C means to hold your upper body in a C shape with pelvis tilted up, shoulders tilted forward at all times; Ten-Hut! means to keep your chest up and shoulders back, like standing at attention throughout; and the 2-second squeeze means to hold for 2 extra seconds at the top of a rep, or the point of maximum muscle contraction.

If the Machines in Our Photos Differ from Those At Your Gym

The machines I've photographed are representative of the most common machines found in a decently equipped fitness center today. Not all gyms will use the exact same machines, but every gym will have machines that correspond to each exercise and body part I want you to work. If you have any trouble recognizing which machine at your gym corresponds to that of an exercise in this book, take the book to the gym and ask an attendant or trainer to show you the comparable machine and its adjustment points. You'll quickly get familiar with it and be on your way.

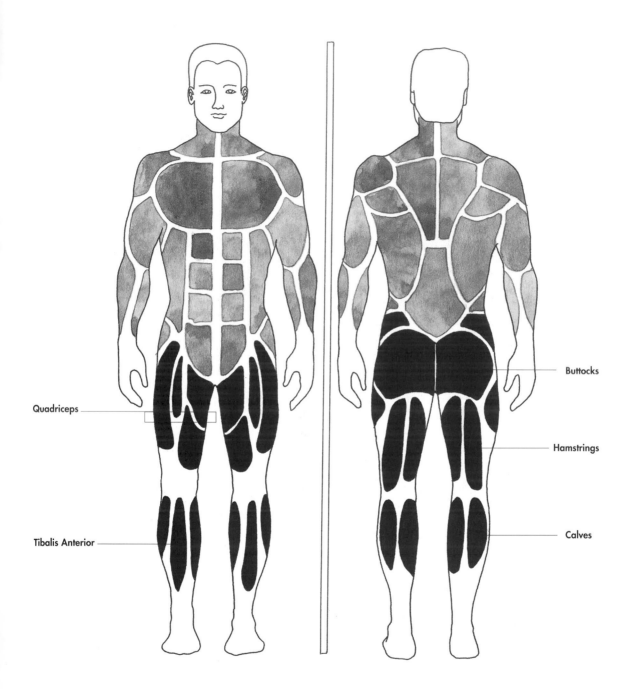

Quadriceps

Tibalis Anterior

Buttocks

Hamstrings

Calves

Legs and Hips

Strong legs and hips are so essential to overall health and appearance, it's no exaggeration to say our lives depend on them. They command our mobility. Their vascular function provides the primary mechanism for blood return to the heart for oxygenation. Older folks with weak legs have blood pooling; puffy, unsightly veins; and restricted movement. Older folks with strong legs have fewer of these problems. Strong legs boost our fat-burning metabolism more than any other group of muscles because of their mass. They maximize our sports ability and minimize injuries. They reinforce our knee and hip joints. And, lest we forget, stronger legs and hips create a shapelier, more youthful appearance for anyone at any age. What better place to begin than with exercises that will give us great, strong legs and hips for life!

Leg Press COMPOUND EXERCISE

There's no more important exercise in any program than the leg press. That's why it's a staple in the majority of my routines. The leg press provides direct stimulus for all of the major muscle groups below the waist, so it's one of the best exercises to warm up your whole body at the start of your workout. It works your thighs (quadriceps and hamstrings) and buttocks (gluteus maximus), and your lower back (erector spinae). These muscles are among the largest in the body, and as they get stronger, they play a major part in boosting your overall metabolism.

STARTING POSITION

- Sit in the seat, your feet waist-width apart on the foot platform.
- Move the seat forward to bring your knees to within 3 to 6 inches of your chest.
- Your hands should be by your sides, gently holding the handles.

EXECUTION

Keeping your buttocks down, gently apply pressure through your heels as you barely begin moving the weight. Continue to slowly extend your legs until your knees are almost straight, but do not lock out your legs. When you reach bottom, don't rest as you start your next rep. Repeat until muscle failure.

TIP

Keep shoulders, arms, and neck relaxed.

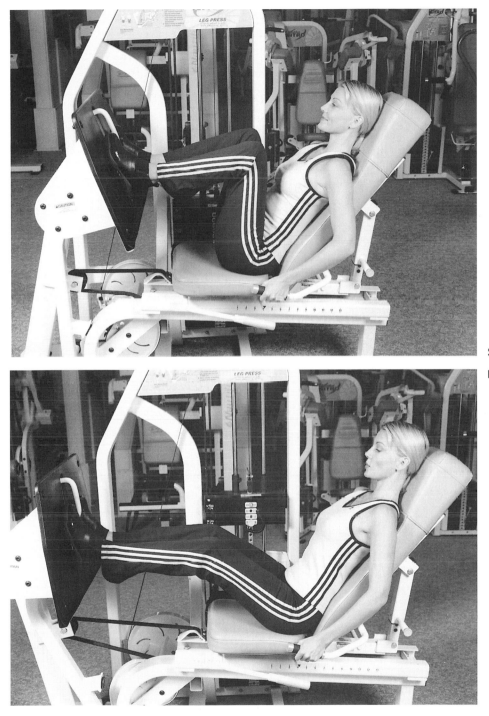

Start

Finish

Hamstring Curl SIMPLE EXERCISE

The hamstring curl is the quintessential exercise for developing and shaping the major muscles at the back of the thigh: the hamstrings. The hamstrings are a group of three muscles: the semimembranosus, semitendinosus, and biceps femoris. Besides their obvious function of bending the knee for walking, running, and some lateral movements, the hamstrings are vital for stabilizing the knee and reducing knee injury.

STARTING POSITION

- Lie face down on the bench.

- Place the backs of your ankles under the roller pads, with your kneecaps just over the edge of the bench.

- Hook your fingers around the handgrips on both sides of the bench. Place your forehead on a 1-inch pad or folded towel for better neck position.

EXECUTION

Slowly bend your knees, bringing your heels toward your buttocks. Do your 2-second squeeze at the top. It's okay for your buttocks to rise off the bench during the positive phase. For greater involvement of your calf muscles, pull your toes toward your knees. As you lower your knees, relax the ankles and let your buttocks sink toward the bench. Repeat until muscle failure.

TIPS

- Keep your head and neck still and straight during this movement.

- Do not twist your body in an attempt to finish a repetition; you may pull a lower back muscle.

- If you have lower back problems this exercise may exacerbate them. If you experience strain or pain, try lower weights and really focus on proper form.

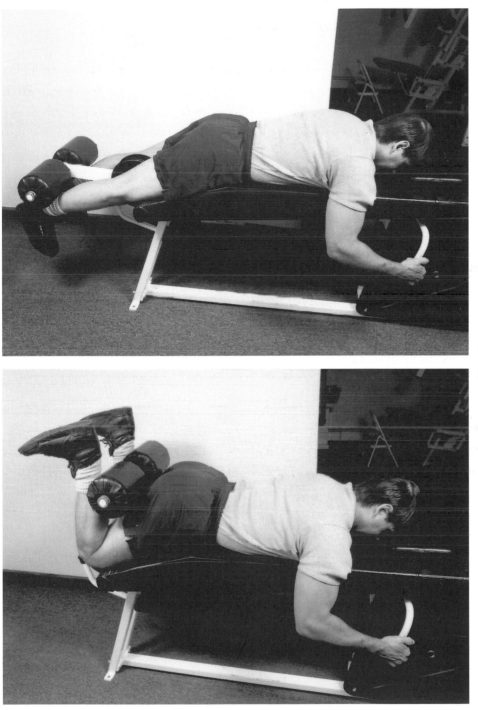

Start

Finish

Leg Extension SIMPLE EXERCISE

The leg extension machine isolates and shapes the upper thigh muscles, which are called the quadriceps femoris, or the "quads." The quads are a large muscle group having four distinct bellies or bodies whose main action is to straighten the knee. They converge into a single tendon that crosses under the kneecap and attaches to the top of the lower leg (tibia). The quads are considered the strongest muscles in the body and together with the hamstrings, add critical support to the knee joint. For this reason, the leg extension is often used in knee rehabilitation. For those with lower back problems, this exercise is the best substitute for squats or the leg press.

STARTING POSITION

- Sit in the seat and bring both legs behind the roller pads of the movement arm.
- Legs should be parallel, not flaring in or out.
- For safety, the starting knee (flexed) position should be at a 90-degree angle. If the machine lacks an angle adjustment, pin the weight stack so your legs start from this point.
- Slide your buttocks rearward until the backs of your knees are a fingerwidth from the front edge of the seat.
- Sit up straight and adjust the back pad so it touches your buttocks.
- Fasten the seat belt, if one is provided, tightly across your hips.
- Place your hands on the handgrips alongside the seat. Lean back.

EXECUTION

Slowly squeeze your legs forward until straight. Do your 2-second squeeze at the top, then slowly lower to the starting position. Repeat until muscle failure.

TIPS

- Keep ankles relaxed.
- During the positive phase gently pull on the handgrips to facilitate full extension.
- Relax neck and shoulders and avoid throwing your head back and forth.

CHEATING POINT

Don't let your butt rise out of the seat to complete a rep.

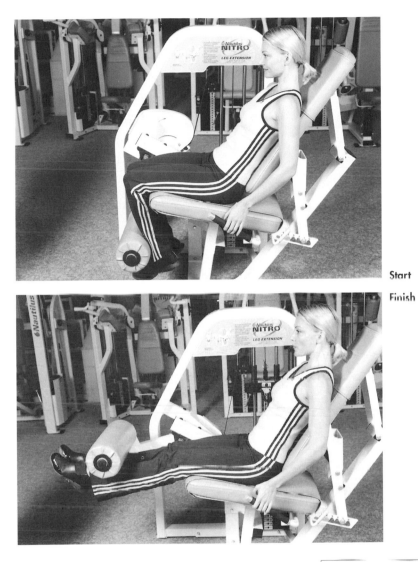

Start

Finish

Cheating point

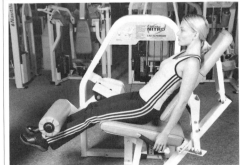

Calf Raise, Machine SIMPLE EXERCISE

The calf raise is an underestimated exercise. A strong calf plays a critical role in walking, running, jumping, and pivoting. Its two major muscles, the gastrocnemius and the soleus, are responsible for bearing nearly all of the body's weight. And the ankle, one of the body's most crucial yet vulnerable joints because it's not surrounded by muscle tissue, gets its chief support from the ligaments, which are attached to the muscles of the calf.

STARTING POSITION

Calf raise machines vary from seated, to standing, to bent-over types. Ask the attendant at your gym to show you the proper starting position in the calf raise machines. Once the balls of your feet are on the foot platform, the execution of all calf machines is virtually the same.

EXECUTION

Lower your heels, letting your calf muscles stretch as far down as possible. Then begin by slowly raising your heels as high as you can. At the top of the motion, do the 2-second squeeze technique. Then gently lower your heels back down to a full stretch without bottoming out or unloading the muscles.

TIPS

- Do not bounce either into or out of the stretch, to keep from hurting the injury-prone Achilles tendon.

- At the top of the motion, visualize trying to stand up on your tiptoes like a ballet dancer.

SPECIAL NOTE

Some standing calf raises require you to lift the weight from pads on your shoulders. I do *not* recommend this type of calf raise machine because of the spinal compression it causes. If your gym only provides this type of machine, I strongly suggest that you use the standing, one-legged calf raise with free weights exercise described on page 120.

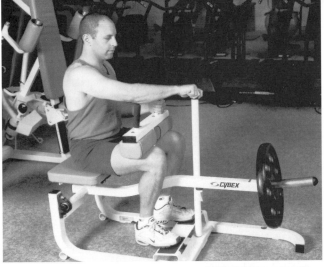

Setup

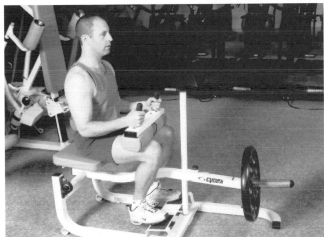

Start

Finish

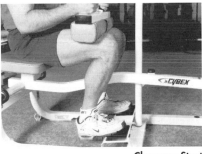

Close-up: Start

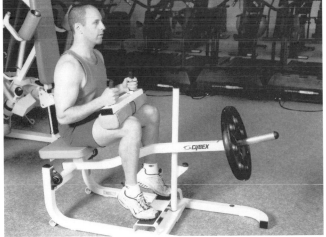

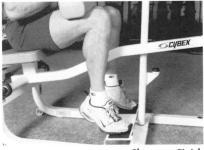

Close-up: Finish

Standing, One-Legged Calf Raise with Free Weights SIMPLE EXERCISE

The standing, one-legged calf raise is one of the few exercises that can be just as effective with free weights as with machines at the gym. It is particularly effective on the large, gastrocnemius muscle because you perform it while standing.

STARTING POSITION

- Place the ball of one foot on a solid raised platform like a stair or a stepstool.

- Hold a dumbbell in the same hand as the foot that is doing the exercise, that is, left hand for left foot.

- Wrap the free leg around the ankle of the working leg, as shown. Steady yourself with the arm that's free, either against a banister or a wall.

EXECUTION

Lower your heel, letting your calf muscles stretch as far down as possible. Then begin by slowly raising your heel as high as you can. At the top of the motion, use the 2-second squeeze technique, then gently lower your heel back down to a full stretch without bottoming out or unloading the muscles. Repeat with the opposite leg until muscle failure.

TIPS

- Do not bounce either into or out of the stretch, to protect the injury-prone Achilles tendon.

- At the top of the motion, visualize trying to stand up on your tiptoes like a ballet dancer.

- Correct amount of weight: the exercise is effective with anything from zero to whatever weight is comfortable to pick up and hold throughout the exercise. Start gradually, then add weight in small increments as your number of reps or time increases.

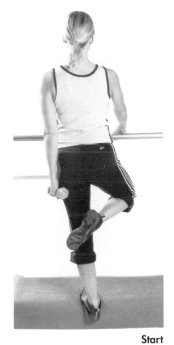

Start

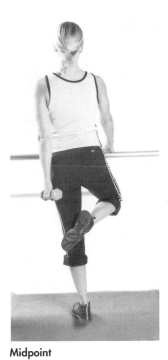

Midpoint

Finish

Close-up: Finish

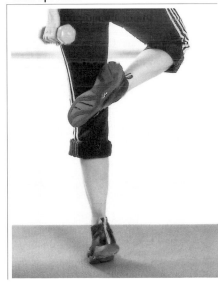

Wall Squat with Ball SIMPLE EXERCISE

The wall squat is another of those home exercises that can give you stimulus and benefit on a par with machines found at the gym. You can even progress the exercise by holding dumbbells at your sides as you get stronger and more advanced. The wall squat mimics the leg press in its involvement of joints, and the muscles it trains.

STARTING POSITION

To best perform this exercise, use a standard 32-inch inflated exercise ball, found at any gym or fitness store.

- In a standing position, place the ball between your lower back and the wall

- Creep your feet forward so that they're about 24 inches in front of you. Keep your back straight and your arms crossed over your chest.

EXECUTION

Slowly begin lowering your buttocks, with the ball rolling along your back, until your thighs are parallel to the floor and your knees are bent at a 90-degree angle. Pause at the bottom for your 2-second squeeze, then slowly start back up. Keep your knees bent at the top, being careful not to lock out. Repeat until muscle failure.

TIPS

- It's important to keep your back moving in a vertical, straight-up-and-down motion, not leaning backward or forward.

- When you start back up from the bottom of the squat, press through your heels—just like with the leg press—not through your toes or the balls of your feet.

- Use rubber-soled shoes, or perform on a surface with traction that won't allow your feet to slide forward and out from under you during the exercise.

- Place a pillow on the floor against the wall, just in case when you reach muscle failure, you need to drop to the floor.

CHEATING POINT

- Remember not to lean back at an angle—keep your torso straight and vertical.

- Don't stand up so high that your knees lock out.

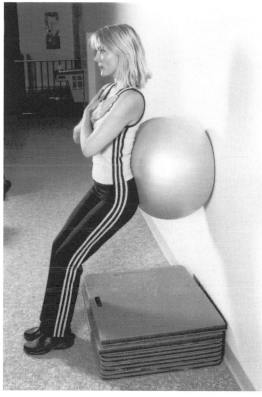 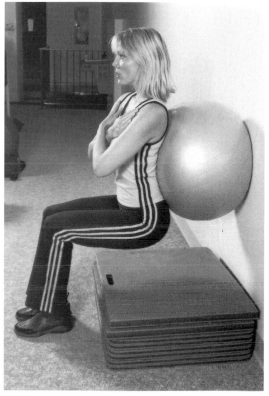

Start   Finish

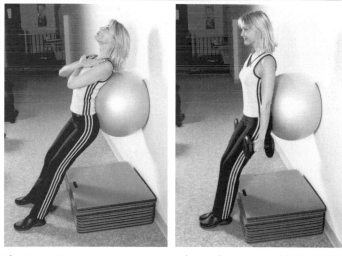

Cheating point   Advanced variation: with dumbbells

Wall Squat, Static Hold SIMPLE EXERCISE

Use this version of the wall squat when you don't have a ball to work with.

STARTING POSITION

- In a standing position, place your back against the wall.

- Let your back slide down the wall and creep your feet forward so that they're about 24 inches in front of you, or enough for your legs to be at a 90-degree angle.

- Keep your back straight and your arms crossed over your chest.

EXECUTION

Hold this position until you reach muscle failure, then exit by slowly sliding all the way down until you're sitting on the floor.

TIPS

- Use rubber-soled shoes, or perform on a surface with traction that won't allow your feet to slide forward and out from under you during the exercise.

- Place a pillow on the floor against the wall so you can sit down on it.

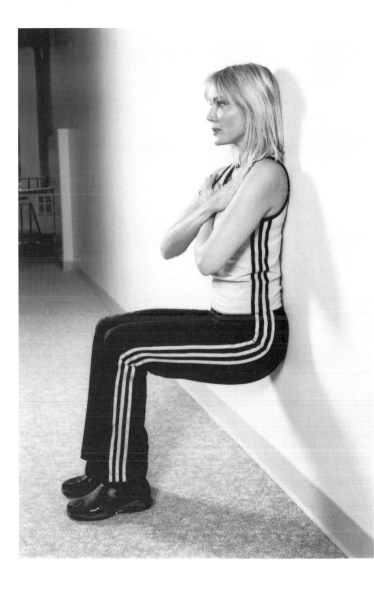

Hip ADduction (Starting Wide, Pulling Legs Inward) SIMPLE EXERCISE

Hip adduction exercises the inner thighs and groin. Strength in this area is important to protect your pelvis, hips, and thighs, particularly in running sports. Groin pulls are among the most painful and persistent sports injuries. Strong, supple muscles in this area help prevent them. For women, this is a particularly important area to strengthen in preparation for childbirth.

STARTING POSITION

- Set the movement arms in position so that when you get seated in the machine, your inner thighs and groin will experience a moderate stretch. This stretch need not be excessive.

- Sit comfortably so that your legs rest on the contours of the leg pads, whether flat or slightly curved. Fold your hands and place them on your stomach.

EXECUTION

Move your legs together all the way, gently touching the pads, using the 2-second squeeze technique when the pads touch. At this point you can even do a little ab crunch while squeezing for maximum effect. Bring your legs back apart, without resting at the bottom of the motion. Repeat until muscle failure.

TIP

Don't tense up your body, don't arch your back. Keep the action smooth.

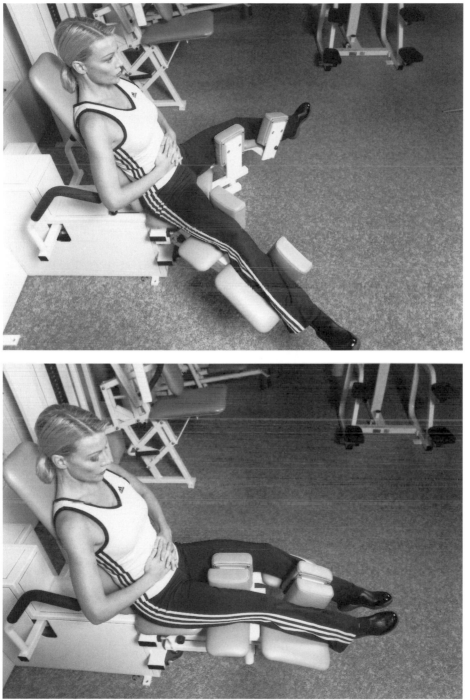

Start

Finish

Hip ABduction (Starting Together, Pushing Legs Outward) SIMPLE EXERCISE

Hip abduction primarily strengthens the muscles of the buttocks, and secondarily, the outer thighs. Strong, shapely buttocks do more than just look good on the beach. Buttock muscles are involved in nearly every movement of your lower body, from walking and running to kicking—even just balancing while you stand. Hip abduction is an especially important exercise to help prevent osteoarthritis of the hip as we age.

STARTING POSITION

- Sit in the machine, placing your legs in the movement arms, adjusting if possible so that the knee pads touch against the lower thighs, just above the knees.

- Knees should be tightly together at the start of the movement.

- If the machine has a seat belt, by all means use it. If the machine has handles, push down on them with your palms, bringing your shoulders, back, and chest up as you start the exercise.

SPECIAL POSTURE

Use the Ten-Hut! chest-up, shoulders-back position during the positive phase—from starting point to legs all the way apart. Relax the Ten-Hut! position on the return phase as you bring your legs back together.

EXECUTION

Begin slowly, smoothly moving your legs apart, holding the Ten-Hut! position with shoulders back. At the top of the motion, when your legs are fully apart, use your 2-second squeeze technique. As you start back to the beginning of the motion, relax the Ten-Hut! body posture. Go into the Ten-Hut! again as you bring your legs back outward.

TIPS

- On hip abduction machines with handles, push against them with your palms; don't pull up on them.

- Remember: Ten-Hut! position going out, relaxed body coming in.

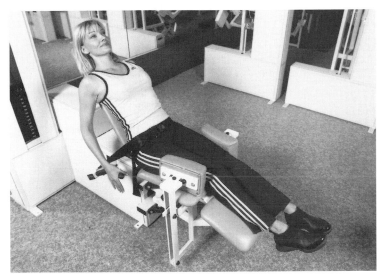

Start

Finish

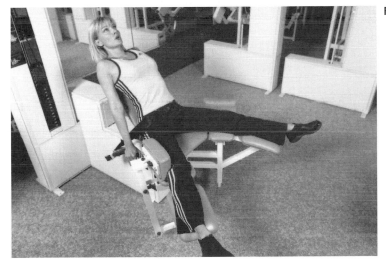

Close-up: "Ten-Hut!"
during positive phase

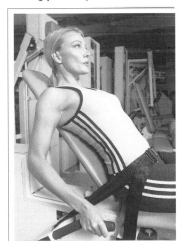

Floor ABduction SIMPLE EXERCISE

This exercise can be substituted for the hip abduction machine when you're at home and/or on the road.

STARTING POSITION

- Lie on your side with your lower arm bent under your head, using your forearm like a pillow.

- Put a pillow between your arm and head if you like.

- Keep your legs very straight, with your knees locked out. Flex your foot so the heel pushes out.

EXECUTION

Lift your top leg upward as high as you can, keeping it straight throughout the movement. Do the 2-second squeeze at the top, then slowly lower your leg without resting at the bottom. Repeat until muscle failure.

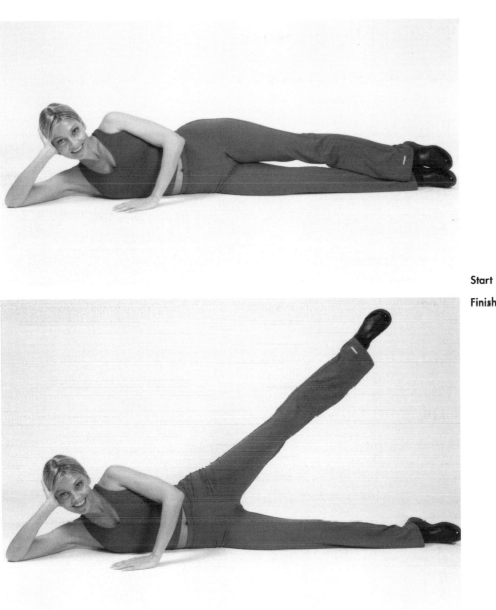

Start

Finish

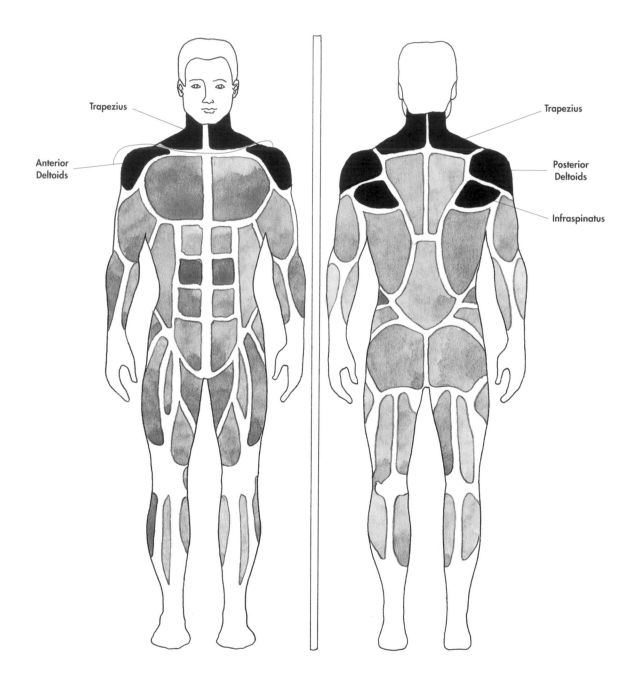

Trapezius

Anterior
Deltoids

Trapezius

Posterior
Deltoids

Infraspinatus

Shoulders and Neck

The shoulder is a remarkable, multijoint structure in which the upper arm (humerus) is attached to the body (thorax), via the collarbone (clavicle) and shoulder blade (scapula). Its complexity allows for an almost universal range of movement (at least eighteen different types), while also providing a strong, fixed point for lifting and pushing heavy objects. There's hardly a physical activity one can imagine—from raking leaves to throwing a baseball—where the shoulder isn't a vital mechanism. But its complexity also makes it prone to a host of stresses, strains, and injuries if not properly maintained with strength and flexibility training. Eleven shoulder-related muscles are involved in moving the arm, collarbone, and shoulder blade through their various ranges of motion, and no single exercise can effectively address them all. But the good news is that so many upper body exercises overlap into the shoulders, you'll cover your shoulder requirements simply by going through each of the routines.

Shoulder Press COMPOUND EXERCISE

The shoulder press provides direct stimulation for the deltoids, triceps, and trapezius muscles. The deltoids are often considered the "quintessential shoulder muscle," a triangular group of three heads that drape over the shoulder coming to a point 3 or 4 inches down the arm. Strong, well-developed delts broaden your shoulders and protect them from injury by acting as a shock absorber that protects the shoulder girdle from impact.

STARTING POSITION

- Adjust the seat or pin the weight stack so that when you place your hands up against the handles, they are even with or slightly above your shoulders.

- Sit back in the seat and tighten the seat belt, if one is provided, securely across your hips.

SPECIAL POSTURE

Hold the Body C position through the entire exercise.

EXECUTION

Slowly push the movement arm up over your head until your elbows are straight. Do not lift your chest out of the Body C position. Then lower the movement arm, and when the weights barely touch bottom, slowly start another repetition without resting. Repeat until muscle failure.

TIPS

- Push equally with both arms.

- Do not strain your neck too far forward in the Body C position. Allow your head to follow the natural curve of the spine.

- This is a great simultaneous abs exercise if you contract your abdominals throughout the entire set.

CHEATING POINT

As you extend your arms to the top, almost everyone goes out of the Body C position and lifts the chest up. Don't be like them. Stay in your C.

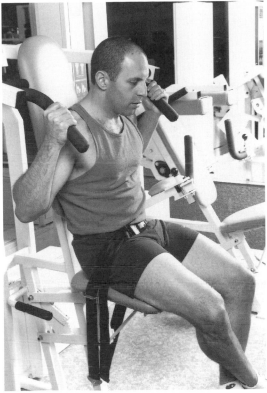
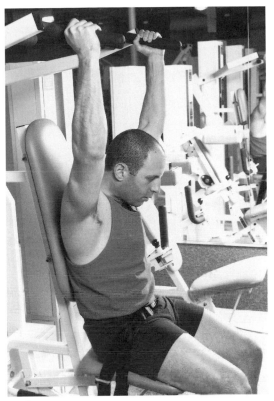

Start   Finish

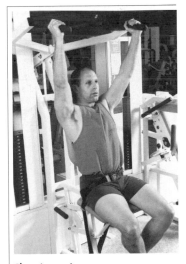

Cheating point

Dip with Machine

The dip is not only a great shoulder exercise, it's a powerful chest and triceps exercise as well. In fact, the dip could just as easily have been included in the chest section as in the Shoulders and Neck section.

SPECIAL NOTE

These instructions apply both to seated dip machines—where your body remains stationary—and to assisted movement dip machines, where you stand or kneel on a moving platform. The assisted movement dip machine is the only counterintuitive machine I know of, because the more weight you put on, the *easier* it is. The weight stack is used to counter your body weight. If you've never been on one of these machines, ask the gym attendant to show you how they work before you use it.

STARTING POSITION

- Position your hands opposite your hips. Your head should be slightly forward and your shoulders should be in their normal posture, not shrugged or rolled.

- On a stationary machine, use your seat belt, if it's provided, and adjust the seat height so that when your elbows are bent to their maximum point of flexion, your shoulders aren't stretched up higher than in a normal posture.

EXECUTION

Hold your body steady as you move the weight upward and downward, keeping your hands opposite your torso. When your elbows are at their most bent position, take care not to let your shoulders shrug upward in order to bend your elbows further. Keep your shoulders in a normal posture alignment throughout, your torso straight. Repeat until muscle failure.

DIP TIPS

You can injure your shoulders if you allow them to stretch or shrug past normal posture at the bent-elbow point of the exercise. Control your motion accordingly.

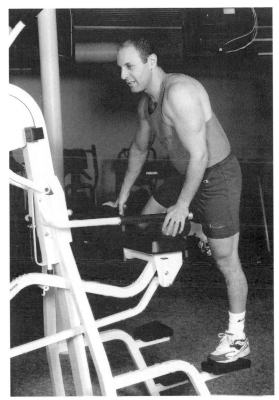

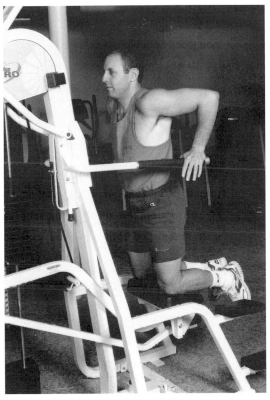

Setup: Assisted dip machine **Start**

Finish

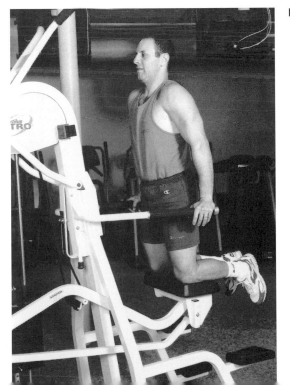

Lateral Raise with Machine SIMPLE EXERCISE

The lateral raise exercise, as the name suggests, involves lifting your arms laterally (from the sides) away from the body until your elbows are approximately even with the tops of your ears. This exercise works all three heads of the deltoids.

STARTING POSITION

- Adjust the machine to align the axis of your shoulders with the machine's axis of rotation. On most machines, this is done with the seat.

- Your arms should be squeezed between your torso and the movement arm. Your hands should hold the handles loosely.

SPECIAL POSTURE

Use the "Ten-Hut!" position throughout.

EXECUTION

Raise your elbows away from your body to a height approximately parallel with the floor. Do your 2-second squeeze at the top. Then lower your elbows until they barely touch your sides and without resting before beginning your next repetition. Repeat until muscle failure.

TIPS

- Keep your head steady.

- As your elbows reach maximum height, be careful not to shrug or raise the axis of your shoulders.

CHEATING POINT

- Push the pads with your elbows. Be careful not to shift the weight to the forearms and wrist to finish a rep.

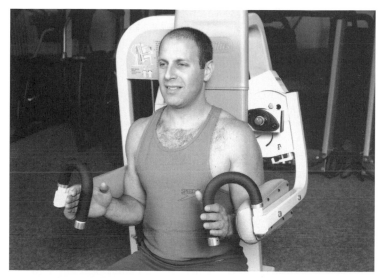

Start

Finish

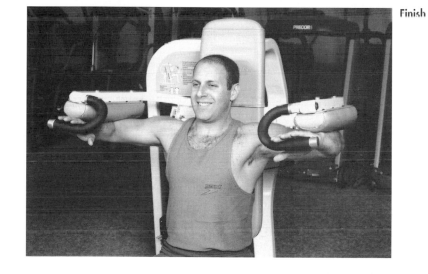

Cheating point

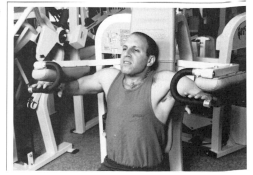

Lateral Raise with Free Weights SIMPLE EXERCISE

STARTING POSITION

- Hold the dumbbells at your sides with your arms straight down, palms facing inward. Stand up in your normal, straight posture.

EXECUTION

Starting with straightened elbows, begin by raising your arms laterally, meaning straight out from the sides, arms still fully extended, using the shoulder as your axis joint. When arms reach a point about a third of the way up, or a foot and a half above your side, begin simultaneously bending your arms at the elbows as you also continue raising them from the shoulders. Keep your wrists and your palms in a fixed position throughout, without swiveling or bending them relative to your arms. As your arms reach their full height—slightly above the shoulder if possible—your elbows should also be reaching a maximum 90-degree bent position at the top of the exercise. Your palms will be facing the floor. Do your 2-second squeeze technique at the top. Lower in the opposite fashion. Repeat until muscle failure.

TIPS

- Be patient in learning and practicing the movement of this exercise. The elbow bend makes the weight seem lighter at the top, placing less stress on the shoulder joint.

- Keep your body as steady as possible throughout.

CHEATING POINT

Don't shrug your shoulders, lean back, or throw your arms to complete any rep.

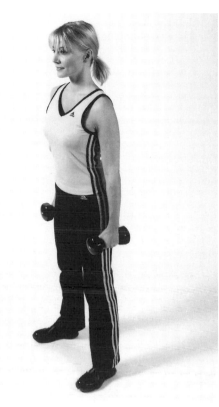 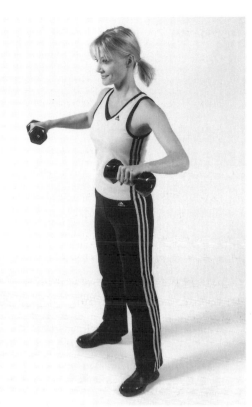

Start **Midpoint**

Finish

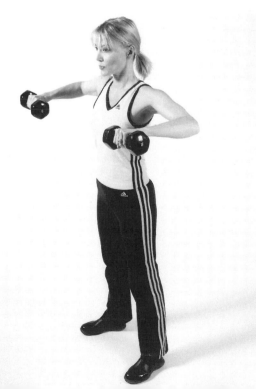

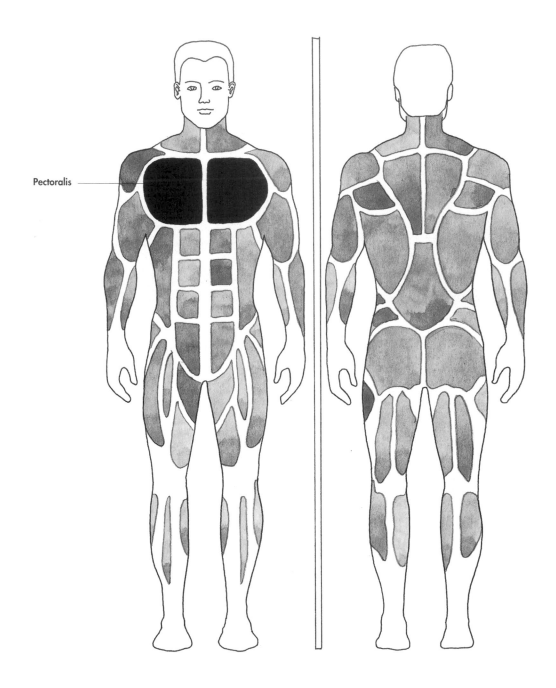

Pectoralis

Chest

You couldn't have the upper body strength you need, or the fit appearance you want, without the pectoralis (pecs) and associated muscles of the chest. They move and protect your arms and shoulders in sports or in any situation that requires a pushing or grabbing motion. A broad chest is the hallmark of a strong man. For a woman, a strong chest and shoulders not only make her look statuesque, they give her a sense of power and confidence when she realizes she doesn't have to go through life with a stereotypical weak and ineffectual upper body.

Chest Press COMPOUND EXERCISE

Chest press is the name given to the exercises that involve extending your elbows (pushing with your arms) and adducting (bringing together) your upper arms. It's one of the most efficient ways to work the upper body in a single exercise. The chest press includes variations, from the seated chest press, the flat bench press, and the inclined bench chest press, all the way to the plain old-fashioned push-up. These exercises target the famous pectoralis major, or pecs, the anterior and middle deltoids, and the triceps. Smaller, stabilizer muscles like coracobrachialis, pectoralis minor, and serratus anterior are worked when you're doing a chest press.

STARTING POSITION—SEATED CHEST PRESS

- Adjust the seat position so the handles are level with your armpits.
- Adjust the handles forward or rearward to give you a moderate shoulder stretch with your elbows slightly behind you.
- Note: You may want to pin the weight stack in this exercise if the handles don't allow adjustment for range of motion, and your beginning shoulder stretch feels excessive.
- Place your feet up on a stepstool to reduce lower back strain.
- Place a rolled-up towel or pad behind your head for extra stability.

SPECIAL POSTURE

Use the Ten-Hut! position.

EXECUTION

From the starting position, without excessive gripping, press your arms forward. Just before your elbows lock out, use the 2-second squeeze technique. Smoothly return to the bottom and without resting, begin your next rep. Repeat until muscle failure.

TIPS

- Do not move your hips during the exercise. Keep them flat.
- Do not arch your back excessively; use a seat belt if available.

CHEATING POINT

Don't lock your elbows or roll over your shoulders to complete a rep.

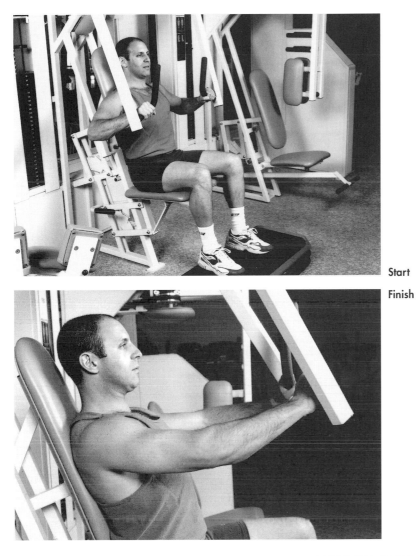

Start

Finish

Cheating point

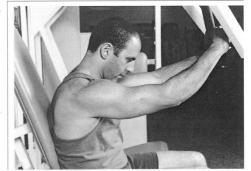

Chest Flye SIMPLE EXERCISE

The chest flye isolates and focuses effort on the pectoralis muscles (pecs) without involving the triceps or excessive shoulder motion. The flye is not only good for variety in your routines, it's good for people with elbow or shoulder problems who want to work the chest without aggravating those areas.

STARTING POSITION

- Adjust the seat so elbows are aligned with the elbow push pads.

- Adjust the location of the movement arms, usually set with pins above both shoulders, so you start and end with your elbows straight out from your sides or with a slight stretch backward.

EXECUTION

Move smoothly until the pads touch. Perform the 2-second squeeze technique at the top of each exercise. Push with your elbows, not your hands.

SPECIAL POSTURE

Hold the Ten-Hut! position—chest up, shoulders back—at all times.

CHEATING POINTS

- Don't push from your hands, push from your elbows.

- Don't shrug your shoulders forward to finish a rep.

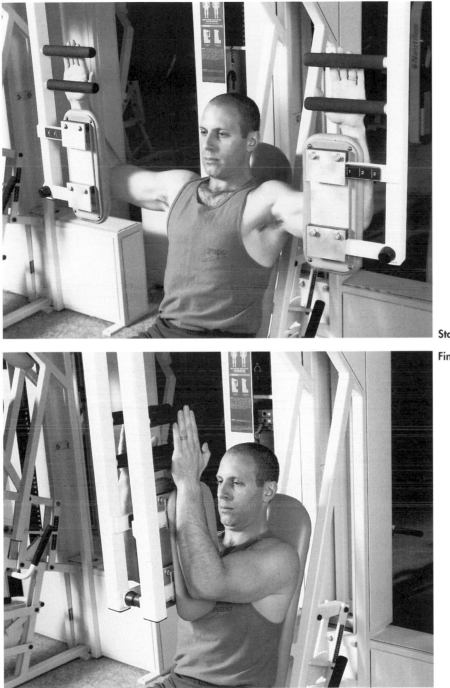

Start

Finish

Classic Floor Push-up SIMPLE EXERCISE

The classic push-up not only works all the muscles that the chest press does, it involves additional groups like the back, the buttocks, and the legs, which are used to keep the body in its correct straight, stable position for the exercise.

THREE TYPES OF PUSH-UP

Push-ups can be performed at various skill levels. Pivoting from the toes with legs straight is the most demanding and effective. Pivoting from the knees on the floor is acceptable for those not strong enough to rest on the toes. For those unable to push upward, even from the knees, "negative-only" push-ups can be performed: you start in the up position, knees on the floor, and simply lower yourself as slowly as possible. Then you get into the up position and lower yourself again.

STARTING POSITION

- Start in the up position, your palms placed a little wider than your shoulders, hands pointing forward, toes on the floor.

- Keep your knees and torso locked so that your body is straight. Keep your neck straight, but your eyes looking down at the floor to prevent neck strain.

- For knee push-ups, relax your legs below the knees, rest on the knees, with all else as above.

EXECUTION

Using the standard Power-of-10 ten-second cadence, lower yourself to the floor. Just as your chest touches the floor, begin pushing back up till your arms are fully extended. Repeat until muscle failure.

TIP

It's acceptable if your buttocks extend upward just a little.

CHEATING POINTS

- Don't dip your chin down to touch the floor ahead of your chest.

- Don't wobble or squirm to push out that last rep.

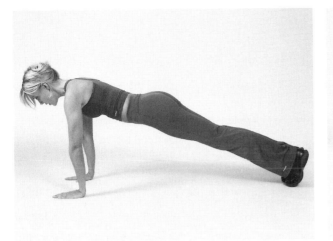
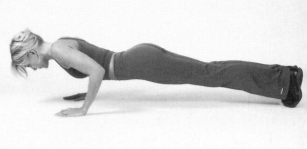

Start: Classic floor push-up   Finish

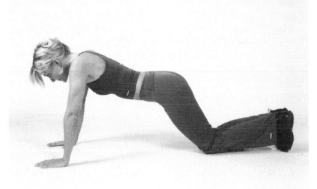
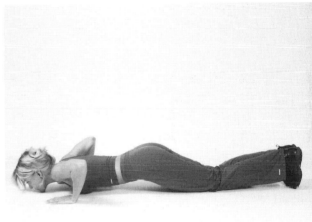

Start: Classic floor push-up from knees   Finish

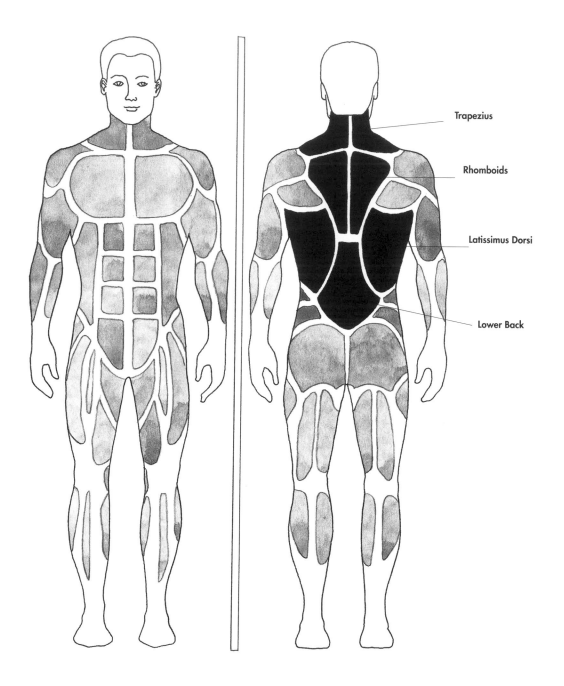

Trapezius

Rhomboids

Latissimus Dorsi

Lower Back

Back

A strong, well-proportioned back is the main factor in building the attractive V-shaped upper body possessed by most fit-looking men and women. Strong back muscles support the shoulders, neck, and spine, and are a major part of any pulling motion involving the arms. Major muscles of the back include the rhomboids, the trapezius, and the rear deltoids. But the largest and most famous back muscles are the latissimus dorsi, or the "lats." Shaped like a giant wing, these dramatic muscles are attached from the middle to the lower part of the spine, then sweep all the way up to the rear of the armpit. When well developed, the lats' V-shaping qualities make it the muscle that made people like Arnold Schwartzenegger and Sylvester Stallone famous.

Lat Pulldown COMPOUND EXERCISE

The lat pulldown—with either the underhand grip (palms toward you) or the over-hand grip (palms away from you) is one of the most effective single exercises for developing the overall upper body. The underhand pulldown simulates the classic "chin-up." The overhand pulldown simulates what used to be called the "military pull-up." The different versions work the forearms and biceps with somewhat different emphasis, and can be alternated for variety. Either way, both exercises give superior stimulus to the chest (pecs), back (lats), rear or shoulder (delts), biceps, forearms, and abdominals—especially if you "crunch" your torso at the end to the positive movement.

STARTING POSITION

- Set the adjustable thigh pad so it's tight against the top of your leg, or buckle your seat belt, if it's provided. With a seat belt machine, you'll need a training partner or spotter to bring the bar down to you so you can start.

- For underhand pulldowns, grip the bar with your hands about shoulder-width apart.

- For overhand pulldowns, grip the bar wider, so your elbows are at about a right angle.

EXECUTION

Starting in the Ten-Hut! position, with your back straight, chest up and shoulders back, gradually start pulling the bar down toward your upper chest. As you move the bar, lower your shoulders and begin to squeeze your abdominals. As the bar reaches your chest, do the 2-second squeeze of your abs and biceps; then reverse direction, allowing your shoulders to go back and your chest to come up as the bar rises back to the top. Just before lockout, with your arms fully extended, begin pulling back down. Repeat until muscle failure.

TIPS

- As you get stronger and use heavier weights, your hands may give out before your back and chest muscles do. Gloves, or the lifting straps sold at most gyms, will help you hang on and increase your time to muscle failure.

- Keep the body steady throughout.

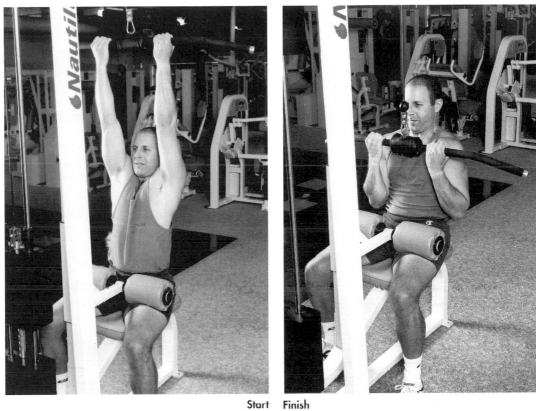

Start   Finish

Compound Row

The compound row is another all-encompassing exercise for the upper body. It's great not only for the lats, rhomboids, and trapezius of the back, and the rear delts of the shoulder, its direct benefits extend all the way to the forearm, the biceps, and triceps as well! As its name implies, it simulates the age-old motion of rowing a boat. For variety, it can be performed with either the parallel grip or an overhand grip like the traditional hold on an oar. Different grips provide a slightly different involvement of the arm muscles between the two exercises.

STARTING POSITION

- Lean your chest against the front pad, with your buttocks pushed slightly away.

- If the movement arms are adjustable, position them so your arms must be fully extended to reach them.

SPECIAL POSTURE

Hold the Ten-Hut! position throughout.

EXECUTION

With either the parallel or the overhand grip, pull your arms back until your shoulders squeeze behind you, then hold for your 2-second squeeze at the top of the motion. Reverse and let your arms out to full extension.

TIPS

- Don't let your shoulders and chest roll forward at the bottom of the motion.

- Keep your elbows tight against your body throughout, especially at the top of the exercise where your elbows are pulled all the way back.

- Try the parallel grip or the overhand grip on different days for variety.

CHEATING POINT

- Remember not to lean back.

- Keep your torso as straight as possible, with your chest against the pad.

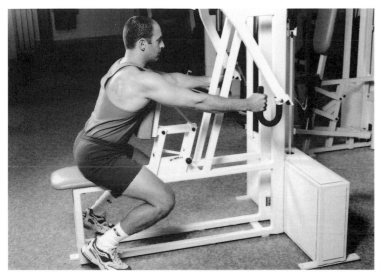

Start

Finish

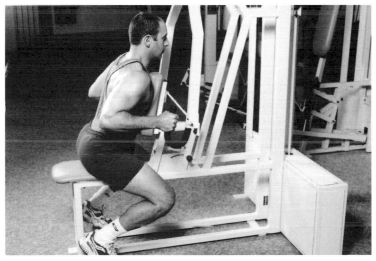

Cheating point

Close-up: Finish (elbows in tight, shoulder blades together)

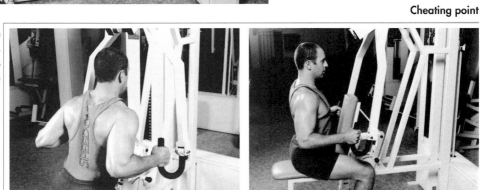

Lat Pullover Machine COMPOUND EXERCISE

I have good news and bad news about this wonderful machine. The good news is it that all by itself, the lat pullover machine provides one of the most thorough, total upper body workouts of any machine you can find. It works the lats and trapezius of the back, the major and minor pecs of the chest, and the delts of the shoulders; not to mention you get a bonus ab workout—all in one exercise.

The bad news is, for some reason, it's rare to find one at a gym these days. My theory is that people simply don't understand what it does just by looking at it, the way they do a chest press machine. They have no idea how beneficial it is, so they skip it. When machines don't get used at the gym, management notices it and they soon get replaced. That's my theory, anyway.

If you see a lat pullover machine at your gym, by all means substitute it into your routines in place of any of the compound back exercises.

STARTING POSITION

- Adjust the seat either up or down so that when you are sitting in the machine, the tops of your shoulders are in line with the machine's axis of rotation.

- Secure the seat belt tightly around your hips. With your feet, depress the foot pedestal, which will bring the movement arm from behind you, into a position where you can reach it.

- Keeping the pedestal depressed, place your elbows or the back of your arms onto the elbow pads. Your hands should be open and lightly resting on the crossbar—not gripping it.

- Releasing your foot pressure on the pedestal, while applying pressure with your elbows, slowly transfer the weight from your feet to your arms on the crossbar. Now let your feet hang freely and begin.

EXECUTION

Pushing with your elbows only—not your hands—begin to rotate the movement arm forward until your arms come around to your sides. Simultaneously rotate your hips upward (pelvic tilt) and "round" your chest downward into the Body C position, in effect, finishing the forward motion with a full ab crunch. Do your 2-second squeeze, then begin your return, rotating your arms backward until your elbows are almost pointing straight up and you feel a comfortable stretch. Release your Body C as you return. Repeat until muscle failure.

To exit the machine, depress the foot pedestal, transferring the weight back to your feet before you let go of the motion arm. Carefully bring the foot pedestal back to its resting position.

TIPS

- Push with your elbows, not your hands.
- Rest your hands lightly on the crossbar, don't grip it, to prevent pushing with your hands.

CHEATING POINT

- Don't lean forward.
- Don't push with your hands instead of your elbows!

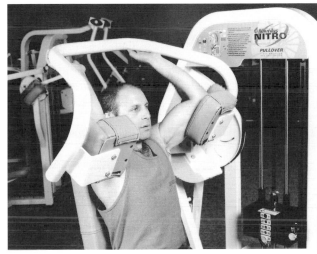

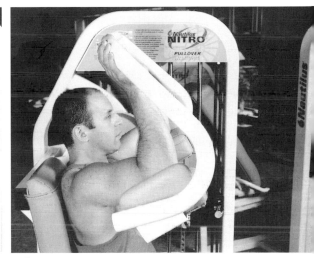

Start Midpoint

Finish

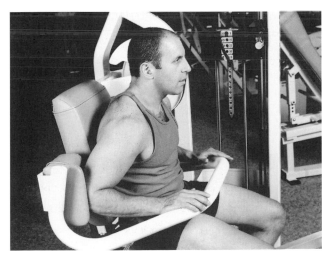

Cheating point

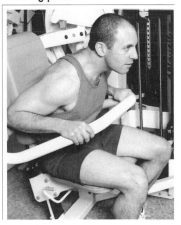

One-Armed Row with Free Weights

COMPOUND EXERCISE

STARTING POSITION

- If you start the exercise with your right arm, place your right foot flat on the floor and rest your left knee on a flat bench.

- Lean forward and support your weight on the bench with your free arm.

- Hold your back and neck straight; avoid rounding or hunching. Look at the floor to reduce strain on your neck.

- Hold the dumbbell with palms facing your body, and keep it in that position throughout.

EXECUTION

Lift your elbows straight up, keeping them close to your body throughout. Hold the 2-second squeeze at the top of the motion, then lower the weight without resting it on the floor until the set is complete. Switch sides and follow the same instructions. Repeat until muscle failure.

TIPS

- Don't lower your head while you're looking at the floor. Keep your neck straight.

- Remember to keep that back straight at all times—don't hunch, roll, or sag.

CHEATING POINT

- Don't arch your back—keep it straight and horizontal.

- Don't tilt your head up or down. Keep it on the same plane as your back.

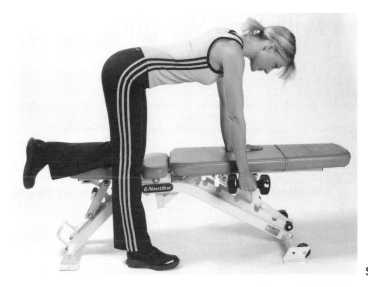

Start

Finish

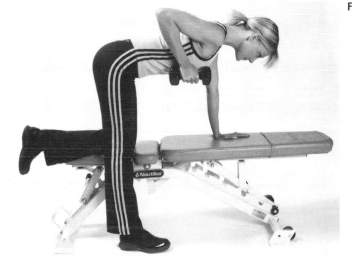

Cheating point

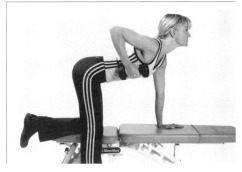

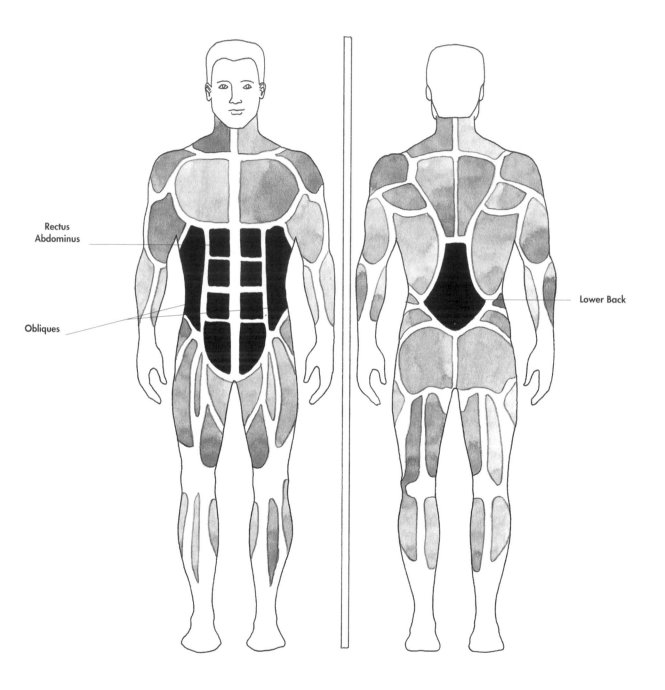

Rectus
Abdominus

Obliques

Lower Back

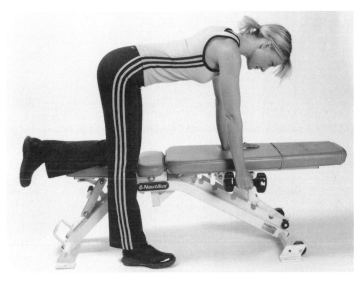

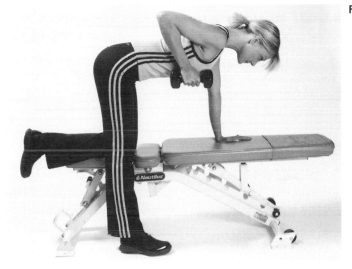

Start

Finish

Cheating point

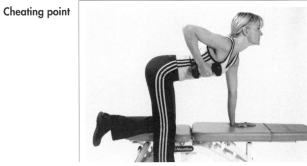

Flat Bench Pullover with Free Weights

COMPOUND EXERCISE

This exercise is great for the lats. It also involves muscles of the chest (pecs), shoulders (delts), and triceps.

STARTING POSITION

- Lie with your upper back on a flat bench, with your body perpendicular or across the pad, knees bent and feet flat on the floor.

- Hold the weight directly above your chin, both arms outstretched.

EXECUTION

Pivoting around the shoulder joint with only a slight flexion of elbow, lower the weight behind your head. Try not to let your hips rise or fall during the exercise. Go back until you feel a nice comfortable stretch, not too far, then reverse and come back up until the weight again is directly above or just slightly ahead of your chin. When you reach muscle failure, just drop the weight behind you. You might want to put a cushion on the floor to drop the weight on.

TIPS

- Keep your hips as stationary as you can throughout.

- Be careful not to overstretch with the weight behind you.

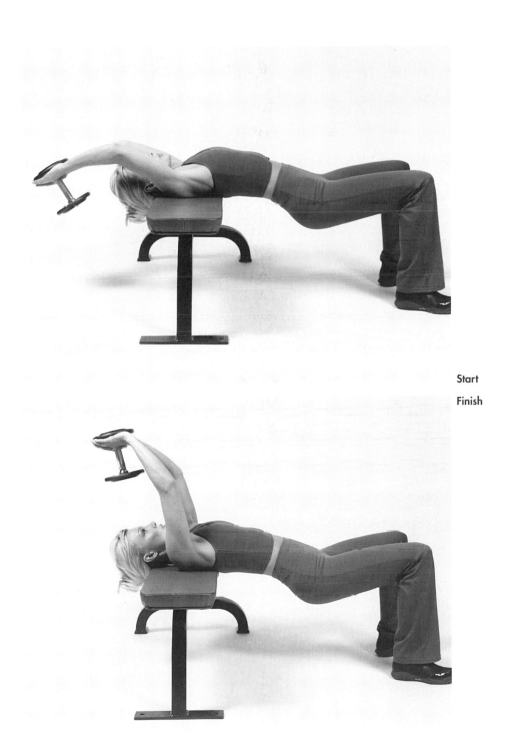

Start

Finish

FLAT BENCH PULLOVER WITH FREE WEIGHTS 161

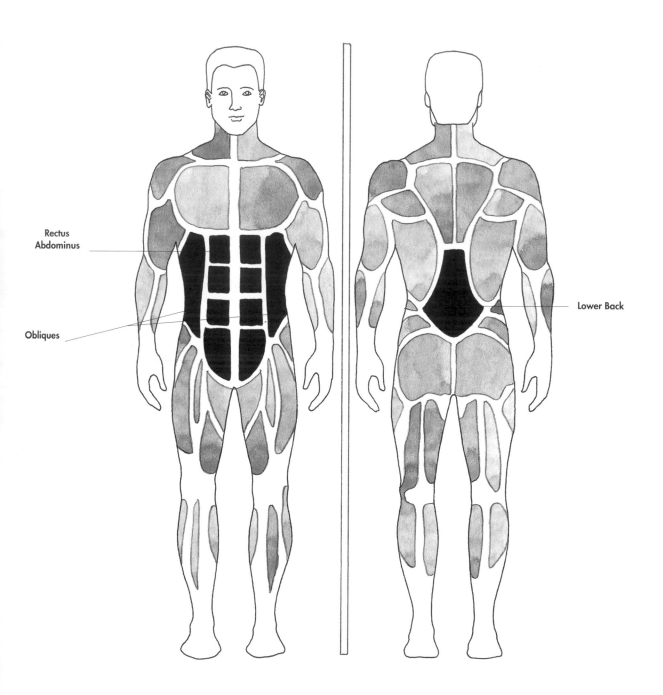

Rectus
Abdominus

Obliques

Lower Back

Core

Your body's "core"—abdominals, obliques, or "side muscles," and lower back—
are crucial to overall body movement and flexibility in sports and in daily living.
They are also critical in protecting your back from debilitating strain, pain, and
injury. A trim, tight midsection enhances anyone's appearance—and greatly
increases your chances of becoming a cover model for a fitness magazine, not to
mention a backup singer for Britney Spears.

One thing to remember about abdominals when using Power-*of*-10 is they're
a muscle like any other in the body. Don't overtrain them, any more than you
would your arms or legs. If you follow normal slow cadences and reach muscle
failure, your abs need 3 to 5 days' rest, as with any exercise. It's also important
to note that a great many of the other exercises in your Power-*of*-10 routine—like
presses and lat pulldowns—have the cross benefit of stimulating and fatiguing
the abs.

There are an infinite number of ab exercise variations. Pick the ones you like,
following the basic principles of form outlined here. With any floor exercise, use
a mat if it makes you more comfortable.

Classic Floor Crunch, Flat or on an Incline

SIMPLE EXERCISE

STARTING POSITION

- Lie face up on the floor, your knees bent upward, feet flat on the floor.

- Place your arms behind your head with fingertips touching your temples, or fold your arms across your chest.

EXECUTION

Focus on lifting with your ab muscles only. Push your back and buttocks into the floor through the entire exercise. Lift your chest until your abs are fully contracted and your shoulders are about 4 to 6 inches off the floor. Imagine a string attached to the center of your chest pulling your torso straight up toward the ceiling. Keep your neck and head straight. Be careful not to tuck your chin into your chest as you lift. If you're doing the exercise with your fingertips touching your temples, keep your arms in the same flat position throughout. Reverse your motion, lowering yourself back to the floor, but stop just before touching your shoulders or head to the floor, and do not rest until you reach muscle failure.

TIPS

- Don't lock your fingers together behind your head. Keep your fingers pointed straight, just touching your temples.

- Arms folded over the chest offer the least resistance. Fingers touching the temples offer more. You can increase resistance even further by holding a weight plate on your chest under your folded arms.

- Using an incline bench adds variety and increases resistance.

- Don't bend at the waist or come all the way up as in an old-fashioned sit-up. When your abs are contracted, reverse your motion.

- Hold a 2-second squeeze at the top.

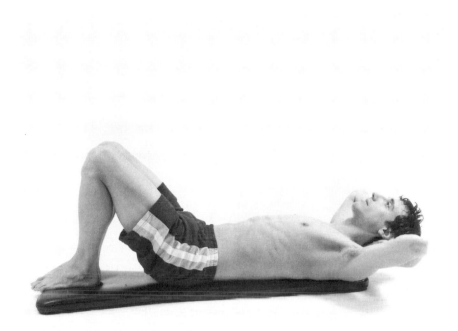

Start

Finish

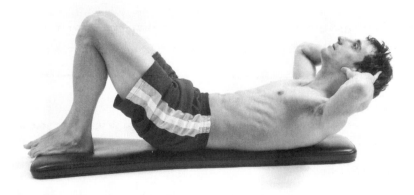

Combo Crunch Simple Exercise

In this exercise, the upper body and lower body move up to meet each other in a jackknife fashion. The knees are bent and raised to meet the torso, which is simultaneously performing a classic floor crunch. This exercise can be more intense than the floor crunch, leading to quicker muscle failure.

STARTING POSITION

- Lie face up on the floor (or floor pad), with legs outstretched.

- Place your arms behind your head with fingertips touching your temples, or fold your arms across your chest.

EXECUTION

The lower body and upper body begin to move simultaneously toward each other like a jackknife. The upper body performs a classic floor crunch, with buttocks and back pressing into the floor throughout. As the chest rises, the knees are simultaneously brought up to a fully bent position, as if to touch the chest. The exercise should be coordinated so the knees and chest will reach the top of their movement at the same time. Then the process is reversed until the legs and torso are flat once again, but neither touch the floor nor rest until the exercise is completed at muscle failure.

TIPS

- Don't lock your fingers together behind your head. Keep your fingers pointed straight, just touching your temples.

- Arms folded over the chest offer the least resistance. Fingers touching the temples offer more resistance.

- Hold a 2-second squeeze at the top.

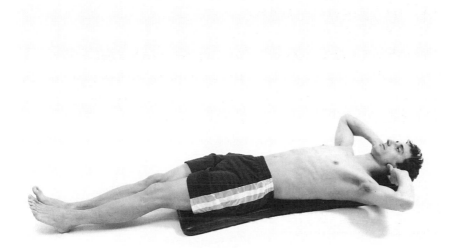

Start

Finish

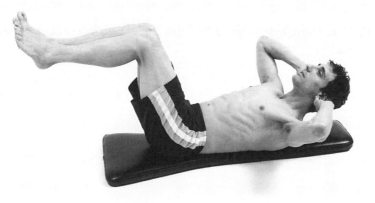

Bent Knee Leg Lifts SIMPLE EXERCISE

This exercise puts your torso through a wider range of motion, providing a stretch for the lower back muscles at the top of the motion.

STARTING POSITION

- Lie flat on the floor, placing your hands underneath your buttocks, palm downward. Your hands stay in this position throughout the exercise.

- Lift your head just off the floor and keep it in that position throughout the exercise.

EXECUTION

Keeping your hands on the floor, begin lifting your legs, simultaneously bending them at the knees as they rise off the floor. Continue pulling your knees toward your chest until they are as close as possible, bending them fully in the process. As you reach the top, let your buttocks and pelvis roll up off the floor until your torso is fully flexed and your abs are contracted to their maximum point. You should feel a moderate stretch in your lower back. Then lower the knees, smoothly and simultaneously extending the legs until they are straight once again. Do not rest them on the floor. Hold your extended legs an inch or two off the floor, then repeat the entire motion until muscle failure.

TIPS

- Keep your back flat on the floor. Don't let it arch upward as you lift or lower your legs.

- Don't lift your head or shoulders—keep your head in a fixed position, just an inch or so above the floor.

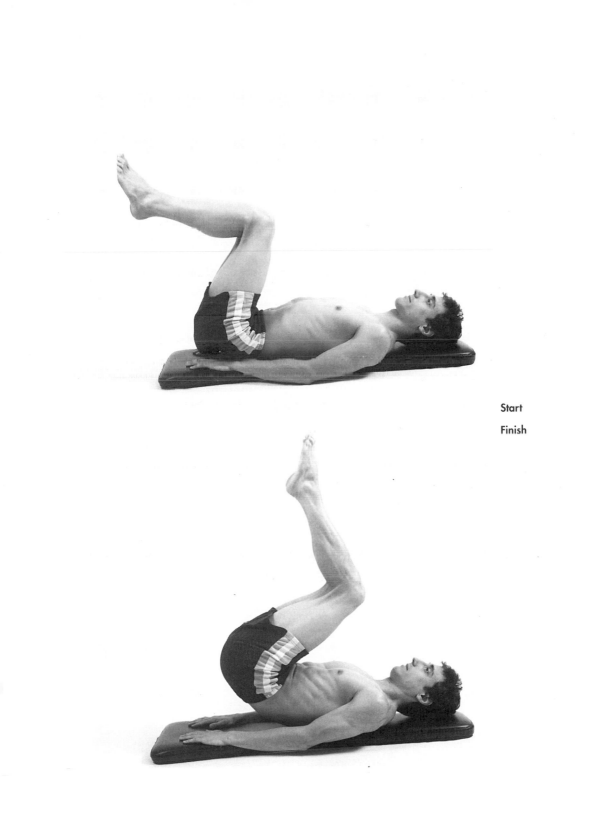

Start

Finish

Twist Crunch for Obliques SIMPLE EXERCISE

This variation of the ab crunch provides greater involvement of the obliques, or the side muscles of your torso.

STARTING POSITION

- Lie in the same starting position as the classic floor crunch with knees bent, feet flat on the floor, back pressed downward, and arms behind your head with tips of your fingers touching your temples.

- Keeping your back flat, let your knees fall all the way to one side, so that your thigh rests on the floor and the other leg rests directly on top. Your torso will be experiencing a yogalike twist.

EXECUTION

Perform crunches in this position, using the same principles, techniques, and tips as the classic floor crunch: press your back into the floor throughout. Don't rest your head at the bottom and don't tilt your neck forward during the motion. Try to raise yourself from the chest. Hold your maximum contraction at the top for your 2-second squeeze, then lower yourself and continue until muscle failure. Switch sides and repeat the exercise.

TIPS

- Focus on your obliques throughout.

- The range of motion is so limited in this exercise, it's okay for positive and negative movements to take less than the normal 10 seconds. Five-second motions are fine—especially if you remember your 2-second squeeze at the top.

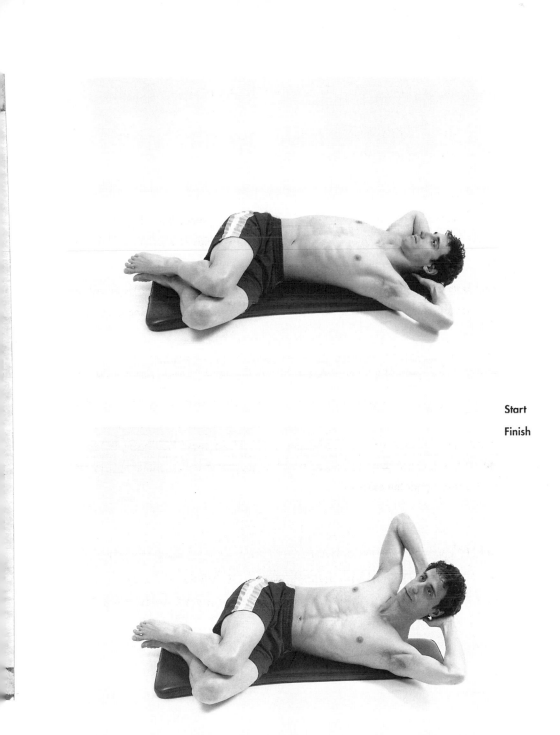

Start

Finish

Side Crunch on Roman Chair for Obliques

SIMPLE EXERCISE

The Roman Chair is great for exercising the obliques through a much wider ranger of motion. The Roman Chair also has the advantage of allowing you to add resistance by holding a dumbbell in your lower hand, or holding a round weight plate under your folded arms if you desire. *Caution: if you have lower back problems, attempt this exercise with caution. If you feel any back pain, stop! Try the previous ab exercises, which have a much more limited range of motion and expose the back to less strain.*

STARTING POSITION

- Position your side on the chair so your lower hip or thigh is on the large upper pad, and the ankle of your opposite leg is tucked under the lower pad, holding you into the equipment. Knees are slightly bent.

- Adjust the height of the upper pad so that it rests on your lower hip or thigh in a way that lets you bend sideways and downward without restriction.

- As in a floor crunch, place your hands either in the fingertips-to-temple position, or in the folded-across-the-chest position.

EXECUTION

Lower your torso straight downward, bending sideways at the waist as far as you can until you reach a slight stretch at the bottom. Then return, contracting your obliques on the upper side, bringing your body up as high as you can. Hold your 2-second squeeze at the top, then continue until muscle failure. Repeat the entire exercise on the other side.

TIPS

- Don't twist your torso. Keep yourself facing in one direction throughout. Keep your neck straight.

- Do not overstretch at the bottom of the motion. You should feel a slight stretch, not pain. If you have lower back problems, be very careful with this exercise.

- Doing this exercise with your arms folded across your chest offers the least resistance. Fingers on the temples offers a bit more. Holding a weight plate on your chest under your folded arms lets you add as much resistance as you want.

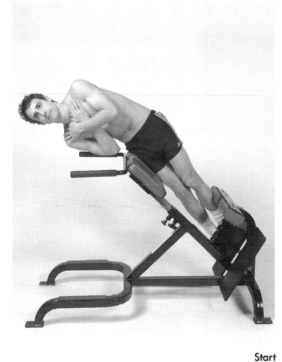

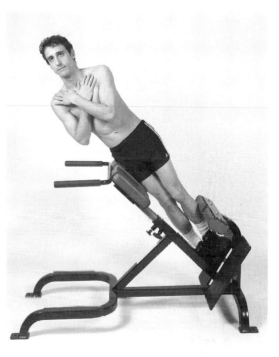

Start   Midpoint

Finish

Advanced variation:
with added weight plate

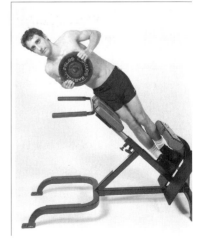

SIDE CRUNCH ON ROMAN CHAIR FOR OBLIQUES

Back Extension, Roman Chair COMPOUND EXERCISE

As with the obliques, the Roman Chair allows much greater range of motion for lower back extensions, plus greater resistance options because you can hold free weights. This exercise strengthens the muscles of the upper and lower back for greater flexibility and injury prevention. It also provides an excellent lower back stretching opportunity at the bottom of the motion. *Caution: if you have lower back problems, attempt this exercise with caution. If you feel any back pain, stop! Try the back extension for the floor that follows, because it has a much more limited range of motion, and it exposes the back to less strain.*

STARTING POSITION

- Position yourself facing downward on the equipment with the large upper pad against your upper thighs or lower hips, and the back of your ankles tucked behind the small, lower pad to hold you into the chair.

- Adjust the height of the large upper pad so that you can bend comfortably at the waist without restriction.

- Fold your arms over your chest, or use the elbows-out, fingertips-to-temple position.

EXECUTION

Lower yourself all the way downward, pivoting at the waist, until you feel a slight stretch. Keep your back and neck as straight as possible. Then start back upward, pivoting at the waist until you're at maximum contraction and you're up as high as you can be. Hold for a 2-second squeeze, then repeat until muscle failure.

TIPS

- Don't round or shrug your shoulders. Keep your back straight.

- Do not overstretch at the bottom of the motion. You should feel a slight stretch, not pain. If you have lower back problems, be very careful with this exercise.

- Doing this exercise with arms folded on the chest offers the least resistance. Fingers on temples offers a bit more. Holding a weight plate on your chest under your folded arms lets you add as much resistance as you want.

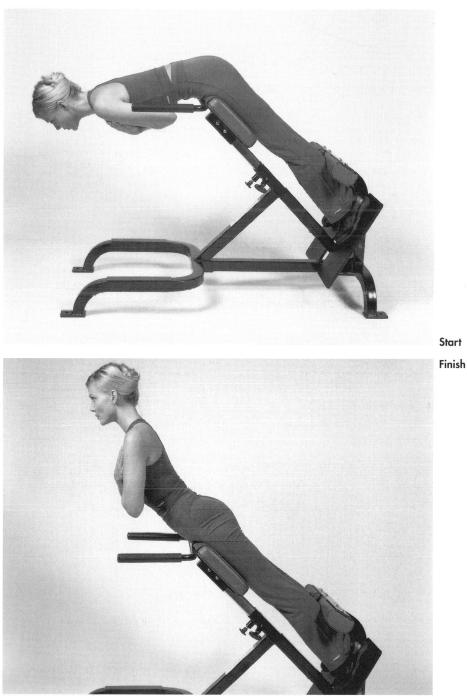

Start

Finish

Back Extension, Floor SIMPLE EXERCISE

STARTING POSITION

- Lie face down on the floor with your body stretched out straight.

- Extend both arms fully along your sides, sliding each hand *under* the upper thigh, with palms facing upward. This will be your pivot point.

EXECUTION

Lift your shoulders and your legs off the floor simultaneously, keeping your knees and neck straight, pivoting at your middle. You should be balancing on your hands and forearms. Hold at the top for your 2-second squeeze, then release downward. Keep muscle tension and do not rest at the bottom. Repeat until muscle failure.

TIP

This exercise has an extremely limited range of motion. It's perfectly acceptable to reduce each motion from 10 seconds to about 5 seconds, especially if you perform your 2-second squeeze at the top.

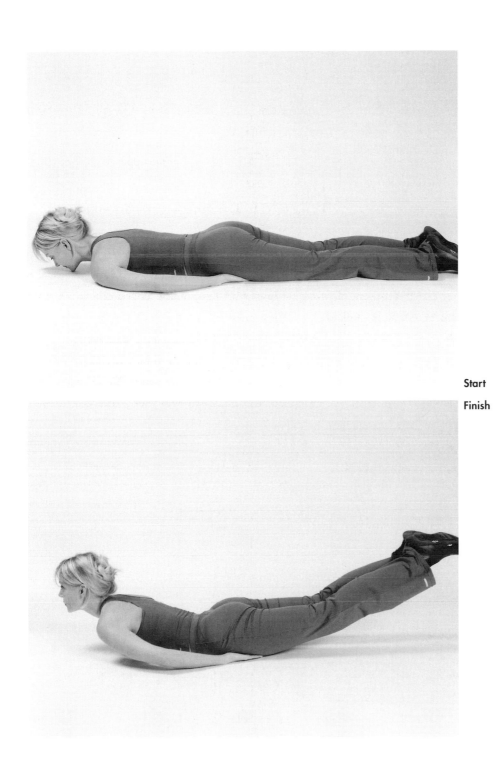

Start

Finish

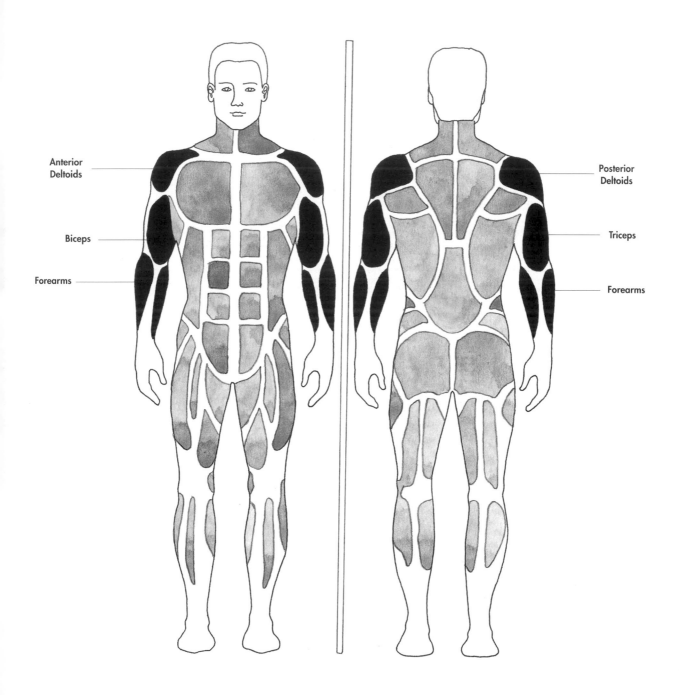

Anterior
Deltoids

Biceps

Forearms

Posterior
Deltoids

Triceps

Forearms

Arms

What can I say about arms? How about, "Try learning the violin without them." Or, "Golf anyone? Without arms?" The uses of the good old arms are too numerous to mention, so I don't have to convince you of their importance and the need to keep them strong and flexible. It's also widely held that lean, well-conditioned arms are attractive to look at, both on men and women. The most famous arm muscle has to be the biceps brachii—the biceps itself—which gives the front of the upper arm its characteristic long, round shape, and that big bulge when we flex it. Helping out are the brachialis, which fits nicely under the biceps; and the brachioradialis, a long, thin muscle that inserts way down on the lower forearm near the wrist, providing extra leverage for arm bending. The brachioradialis also provides the outer contour of the upper forearm, and helps to supinate the wrist, or turn it upward. Other flexors and extensors in the forearm move the hands and fingers and give us our grip. The triceps is probably the arm's second most famous muscle—the one that forms the back of the upper arm and opposes the biceps. It's used in any motion that pushes or extends the arm. Women especially should be reminded that since muscle is more compact than fat, strengthening the biceps and triceps will generally make you look leaner, not cause you to bulk up.

Biceps Curl with Machine SIMPLE EXERCISE

The biceps curl isolates and strengthens the muscles that serve to bend (flex) the elbow. The biceps curl is one of the exercises most commonly performed with dumbbells and barbells. The advantage to the machine, however, is that it eliminates cheating tendencies and provides more uniform, constant resistance through the entire range of motion.

STARTING POSITION

- Place your elbows shoulder-width apart and in alignment with the machine's axis of rotation.

- To avoid hyperextension of the elbows, pin the weight stack up and/or adjust the seat height so that your shoulders are approximately 6 inches above your elbows.

- Your feet should be placed firmly on the floor or on the machine's foot pad to prevent your hips and buttocks from sliding forward.

SPECIAL POSTURE

Maintain the Ten-Hut! position.

EXECUTION

Start the exercise with your arms in the straightened but not hyperextended position. Slowly squeeze your biceps and start to bend your elbows. Without gripping the handles too tightly, and keeping your wrists straight, bring your palms up as close to the front of your shoulders as possible. Do your 2-second squeeze at the top, then lower the bar to the starting position. Without resting at the bottom, slowly start back up. Repeat until muscle failure.

TIPS

- Keep your torso vertical during the exercise. Try not to lean back during the positive phase and don't lean forward during the negative phase.

- Do not bend your wrists.

- Keep the Ten-Hut! position and resist the temptation to shrug your shoulders.

- Make sure your elbows stay in line with the axis of rotation; do not let them slide to and fro.

Don't squirm in your seat, or move your body under the bar to grind out the last rep. Hold your form.

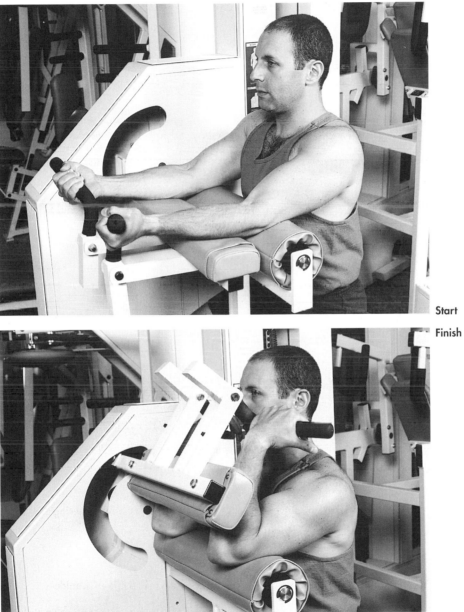

Start

Finish

Biceps Curl with Free Weights
(EZ Curl Barbell or Dumbbells) SIMPLE EXERCISE

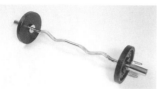

EZ curl barbell

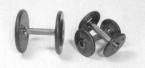

Dumbbells

STARTING POSITION

- If you're using an EZ curl barbell, hold it with an underhand grip and your hands approximately 5 inches apart. With dumbbells, also use the underhand grip and allow the ends to touch.

- Stand 12 to 18 inches in front of and facing *away* from a wall. Lean your lower back against the wall. The rest of your back should be off the wall. Your head and neck should be straight. Your feet should be waist-width apart.

- Press your elbows into your lower ribs and *keep them there*. Permit your arms to stretch downward into the fully extended, starting position.

EXECUTION

Slowly start to raise the EZ curl barbell or both dumbbells, keeping your elbows tucked into your ribs. Halfway through the range of motion, lean forward, allowing your shoulders to round while flexing your elbows as much as possible. Do your 2-second squeeze when you reach the *maximally* flexed (bent) position at the top of the motion. Make *doubly sure* your elbows stay pressed into your sides, or else you will inadvertently rest. Then lower your arms while gradually straightening your torso and bringing your shoulders back. When you return to the fully extended starting point, start another repetition slowly and smoothly. Repeat until muscle failure.

TIPS

- Don't let your body sway back and forth. Keep steady. It's fine if you want to bend your head slightly to watch your hands.

- Don't bend your wrists.

CHEATING POINT

- Don't contort your body or "get under the bar" to dig out the last rep.

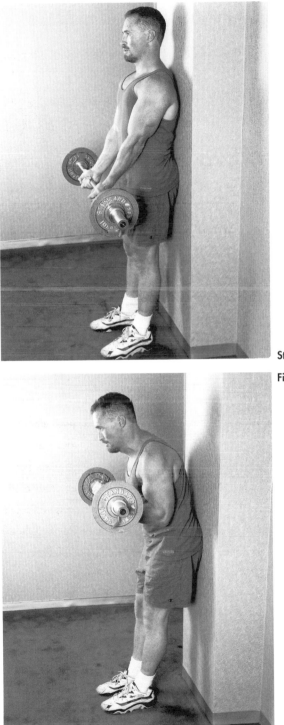

Start

Finish

Concentration Curl with Free Weights

This exercise is performed with dumbbells. It is excellent for isolating the biceps.

STARTING POSITION

- Sit on a bench with your feet wide apart.

- Press the elbow of the arm holding the dumbbell against the inside of the knee on that side. Rest your opposite elbow on the top of your thigh on that side.

- Your chest and head should bend forward. Look at the ground.

- Start with the weight close to the floor, with your arm in the extended position.

EXECUTION

Holding your body steady throughout, lift the weight all the way up to the point of maximum arm bend, or flexion. Do your *best* 2-second squeeze at the top of the motion. Lower the weight slowly, without resting at the bottom. Keep your working elbow locked securely against the inside of your knee throughout. Repeat until muscle failure.

TIPS

- Don't bend your wrists. Don't squirm in any way.

- The better your 2-second squeeze, the better this exercise.

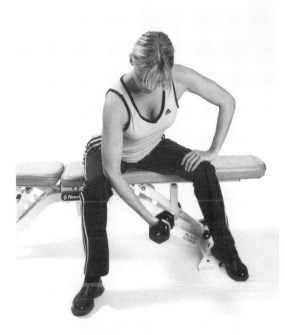

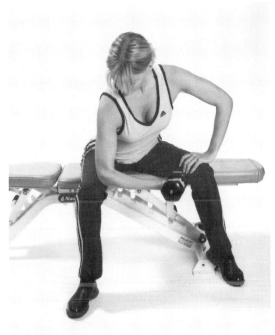

Start   Midpoint

Finish

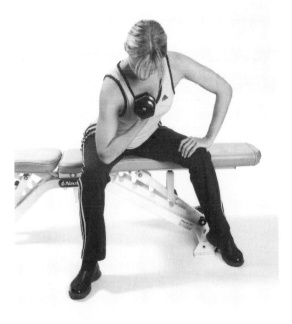

Triceps Extension SIMPLE EXERCISE

This is one of the best pure triceps isolators there is. At most gyms, there are several handle types available for you to snap onto the pulling belt or cable. I recommend using the rope because it's easier at the bottom to really extend your elbows, and puts less stress on your wrists.

STARTING POSITION

- Stand straight or, if a back pad is provided, lean back slightly to touch your shoulders against it. Your feet should be comfortably apart.

- Grab the rope, keeping the elbows tight into your sides at all times.

- Start with the rope in the up position, high enough so that you give yourself a full range of motion from top to bottom, but don't lift your elbows up from your sides.

EXECUTION

Keeping your body stationary at all times, head and neck straight, begin pushing down the rope with your triceps alone. At the bottom and full extension, do your 2-second squeeze, then let the rope back up until you reach your original starting point at the top of a full range of motion. Without resting, repeat until muscle failure.

TIPS

- Focus everything on your triceps. Do not hunch your shoulders or bend your chest down to force out a last rep. Keep your head and body stationary.

- Keep your wrists locked in one position throughout.

- Keep your elbows in one spot, tight to your body, imagining they're a fixed axis. Don't let your elbows rise up and away from your body at the top of the motion.

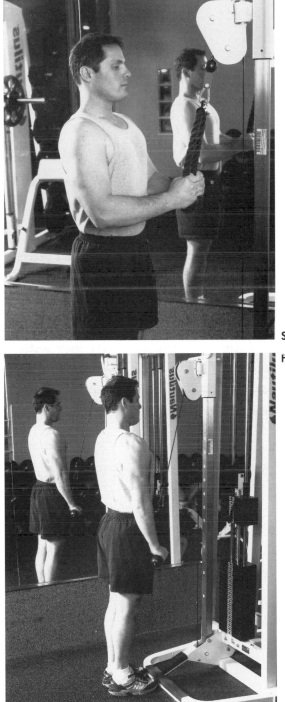

Start

Finish

AFTERWORD:
A WHOLE NEW WORLD

It's always amazed me, the power we have to change our whole world simply by changing one thought, adjusting one attitude, looking at one thing in a new way, or deciding to take one small step in a new direction.

When I was a teenager, if you asked me to name the cruelest form of abuse, I would have said *yard work*. Every Saturday, my father would wake me up at 8:00 A.M. (that's the same as 5:00 A.M. in teenager time) to mow the lawn, rake the leaves, pull weeds, and till the garden while all my friends were heading to the beach. As much as I hated it, my dad loved it, smiling and whistling away, until one day I demanded he explain how anyone but a lunatic could enjoy such boring, dirty work. And he said, "Son . . . the fantastic thing about gardening is that for the cost of a little sweat and exercise, you get to see big, positive changes in your world, very quickly, *every time*. There's nothing else like it. One hour of planting shrubs gives you a whole new landscape. Weeding the gardens gives you a sense of order and precision. Almost every other one of life's endeavors is a compromise between risk and reward, good and evil. But not yard work. Everything you do in your garden is immediately, and obviously, *good*. Now go over there and remove that hornet's nest."

Believe it or not, I began to appreciate our time together after that, and the big changes we made every Saturday. My world got better, just by redirecting a single, simple thought.

The biggest revelation in my professional life is that my dad was wrong when he said "there's nothing else like it." There *is* one other activity where you get to see big, satisfying changes more often than most things in life. Where everything you do is positive. Where you can literally change your physical and mental world, just by deciding to. And this one comes without raking leaves.

I bet you can guess what it is.

There is no higher-profit, lower-risk investment on the planet than simply deciding to be one of the fit people. Anybody can achieve its riches, just by saying the word "yes."

You get better health, you get more beauty, you get more energy, you get more endurance, you get more strength, you get more flexibility, you get more longevity, you get more desire to do things, you get more confidence, you get more self-esteem, you get more positive response from others, you get more opportunities, you get more resilience, you get more success.

I've spent my professional career refining, testing, and perfecting a fitness program that can eliminate the time constraints, injuries, and excuses so that many more people will take the first step, experience success, and so on to a whole new life. I've found the solution and now so have you.

A rich new world of fitness is more than a promise, it's the *guarantee* of Power-*of*-10. Choose to be one of the wealthy.

FORTY OF MY FAVORITE SNACKS

There is an infinite number of creative combinations you can make with good food. These are a few of the snacks and minidesserts that I like to eat, and that I like to make because they take about 1 minute each to prepare.

1 String cheese and whole wheat crackers

2 Low-fat plain yogurt, berries, and low-sugar, whole grain cereal

3 Natural peanut butter and whole grain crackers or flatbreads

4 Whole wheat flour graham crackers and skim or soy milk

5 1 ounce dry-roasted/ unsalted nuts (almonds, cashews, walnuts, soy nuts)

6 1 hard-boiled egg and portion of raw veggies

7 1 serving whole grain, low-sugar cereal with berries and skim or soy milk

8 1 sushi roll (6 pieces), any kind

9 1 multigrain waffle with ½ cup berries and 1 tablespoon *real* maple syrup (less sugar than honey)

10 1 to 1½ cups lentil- or bean-based soup

11 1 to 2 ounces smoked salmon on 1 slice black bread with 1 teaspoon low-fat cream cheese

12 4 to 6 oz. low-fat cottage cheese with ½ cup fruit or ½ banana

13 Raw vegetables and low-fat yogurt dip

14 ½ ounce baked tortilla chips, 1 ounce low-fat jack cheese, and salsa

15 Lisa's snack mix—½ cup whole grain cereal, ½ ounce nuts, and 1 to 2 tablespoons raisins or currants

16 1 mini whole wheat pita and 1 to 2 tablespoons hummus

17 Portion of raw vegetables dipped in hummus

18 8 to 10 large steamed/grilled shrimp and 6 to 8 olives

19 Scrambled egg with salsa and slice whole wheat toast (also my favorite breakfast)

20 ½ banana and 1 tablespoon natural peanut butter

21 1 apple and 1 tablespoon natural peanut butter

22 3 ounces tuna packed in water, 2 tablespoons whipped low-fat cottage cheese, and 3 to 4 Wasa crisp breads or whole grain crackers

23 1 to 2 ounces low-fat cheese melted on 1 slice whole grain bread

24 1 block baked tofu or soy cheese (cheese substitutes) with 1 mini whole wheat pita

25 Turkey wrap—2 to 3 slices fresh turkey, wrapped in romaine lettuce leaf with mustard or hummus

26 White meat chicken wrapped in lettuce and slice of tomato with 1 teaspoon low-fat mayo

27 2 or 3 canned sardines on a whole grain cracker

28 ½ cup low-fat ice cream, plain or with berries and crushed nuts

29 ½ cup low-fat frozen yogurt with berries and crushed nuts

30 Microwaved "baked" apple with cinnamon and 1 teaspoon honey (optional)

31 Mixed berry parfait—1 to 1½ cups berries layered with low-fat yogurt, sweetened with honey or maple syrup

32 Chopped hard-boiled egg and 3 ounces tuna with 1 teaspoon low-fat mayo on a whole wheat pita

33 1 tablespoon natural peanut butter and celery sticks

34 A cup of fresh fruit salad

35 2 turkey breast roll-ups, made from 1 slice turkey, 1 thin slice low-fat cheese, and mustard or a smear of low-fat mayo or low-fat Russian dressing

36 One serving of soy chips

37 A big bowl of steamed broccoli or any green vegetable with 1 tablespoon olive oil, garlic, salt, and pepper

38 Meal replacement shake with water. My favorite brands are Met-Rx, Myoplex, and Apex. Look for shakes with low or no added sugars.

39 Meal replacement protein bars. My favorite brands are any with low carbs and at least ⅓ protein by weight.

40 Whey protein shake with fresh juice or skim milk and berries

Power-*of*-10 is really amazing. It's all anyone needs to be in fabulous shape and lead an active lifestyle. Nature gave us these great muscles to use them, to be active and dynamic, not to let them atrophy by disuse and sitting around. Power-*of*-10 lets people achieve the physical potential we were all meant to have, because no matter where you live or what your schedule's like, there's time for you to work out completely, once-a-week in less than 25 minutes, with this superefficient form of exercise. Take it from a former weight lifter who didn't believe that the fastest results can come by slowing down with Power-*of*-10.

Keri Shukat age 29

PRE-K TEACHER

She Turned Endless Hours in the Gym Into 15 Minutes, Once a Week—and the Best Shape of Her Life . . .

I can't tell you I've ever really been overweight, even though I love junk food. But when I got into my twenties, things started to change. I was getting "less thin" than in high school. It was time to join a gym and get serious about exercise. I started doing every-

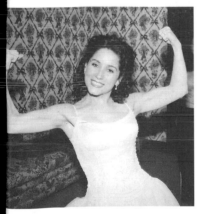

thing—lifting weights, cardio, classes—following the whole program. But as hard as I worked, I never really saw the difference I wanted. I was frustrated and a little fed up with the hours on end I was spending in the gym.

Of all people, my mother had started training with Adam and told me it was the answer. So I gave it a try. At first, I had no idea what to expect with Power-*of*-10. I thought I was just going to see a personal trainer like any other. After one workout, I realized this wasn't like anything I'd imagined. It was intense, different, yet it felt great. The feeling of being totally spent was almost like a rush. I was hooked. You walk out of the workout feeling such a sense of accomplishment, yet it's only lasted 15 to 20 minutes! I never dread going like I used to at the regular gym. I can't wait till it's my once-a-week workout day. And since I'm so competitive, I'm always trying to beat my last TUF—time until failure.

I'm now in the absolute best shape of my life—better than when I was a teen. I don't

Matt Rottino age 36

HIGH SCHOOL TEACHER

He Tried Power-of-10 on a Dare . . .

My story is simple. I was a regular weight lifter. Five days a week, 2 hours a day, including cardio. When you lift that much, it's like an addiction. Even though you don't necessarily like spending your whole life at the gym, you feel like it's just something you have

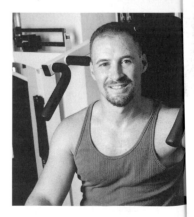

to do every day, like brushing your teeth. I met Adam a few years ago and he told me about his method. I was sure there was no way lifting once-a-week could produce the same results as 5 times a week. How could it? But Adam insisted. He dared me to try it just once. I did and the rest is history.

The first thing I noticed was that the intensity was greater, even though the workout was so much shorter. I was amazed, but I quickly began getting stronger and stronger, more defined than ever. When I switched to

once-a-week after a few months, the results were even more dramatic! Believe it or not, I now actually rest as many as 10 days between workouts and I'm in the best shape of my entire life. The best thing for me is that *I was able to stop doing cardio and aerobics completely*. That's the one thing that I always had to force myself to do, but not anymore. And I haven't had an injury from a workout since I started, over 4 years ago.

worry about pounds on the scale because I've replaced soft fat with lean muscle. I never get any injuries with Power-*of*-10. I can lift 410 on the leg press stack (and I only weigh 97 pounds)! That's a lot for a small person like me. And when I look at my stomach these days, for the first time in my life, I smile.

Jeff Daly age 53

MUSEUM DESIGN DIRECTOR

He Finally Got Off the Overweight Roller-Coaster—at 51

I've been fighting with my weight since I was a teenager. When I hit middle age, I had to admit I was really losing the battle. For a while, I signed on with one of the big city health clubs and did their whole program with a vengeance. Weight lifting, cardio, diets at least 4 days at the gym every week. I got things under control, but it was just too hard to keep the routine. I was always busy, always running from work, always pressured—so the outcome was inevitable. I skipped the gym one day. Then the next. Then a week went by. Then it was hard to go back. Then I was finished. I had quit and I didn't have the energy to get restarted. I gained the weight back so fast I felt like a real sludge. I got up to 223 pounds and I was miserable.

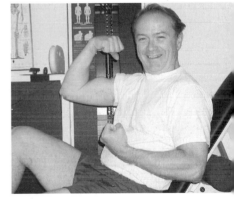

Then someone I knew at the museum told me about this great nutritionist. When I visited her, she was adamant about one thing if I wanted to be her client—I had to exercise—and the program she was recommending turned out to be Adam's. She said her other clients were having amazing success with it and it was accelerating their weight loss. I couldn't believe the claims she was making about it—that you could do your whole routine in one brief session a week—but I trusted her enough to call Adam's studio and give it a try.

It's hard to believe, but in just the first Power-*of*-10 workout, I decided this was it! I knew immediately it was no gimmick or fly-by-night concept—not by the way I felt walking out of the fitness center the first time. It was more like I crawled out. After only 20 minutes, I felt like every muscle fiber in my body had been maxed right out. I'd never felt that way after any workout I'd ever had. It was an intense, but great feeling. I started twice a week. Within a month, the strength was coming back into my legs and upper body. I stuck with the nutrition plan, too. I knew I was getting in shape underneath all my fat, but what I didn't know until a few months later was that I was getting a whole new body! Today, I feel like I'm 18 again. I look in the mirror now, and I can't believe that's the same body that was overweight in my twenties. I have a strength and shape and overall sense of fitness that I've never experienced. I'm off the weight roller-coaster for life because I've found the way to keep my body under control, with a program that's amazingly easy to stick with.

Eventually, I went back to doing the kinds of aerobics I like, a few times a week. I ride my bicycle in the warm weather for the fun of it now. That's the key point—for the fun of it, not because there's any pressure. If I don't do cardio or aerobics one week, who cares? I get all the exercise I need from Power-*of* 10, anyway.

I tell everyone who's interested about Power-*of*-10, but one thing I've learned is to do a soft sell because it sounds so unbelievable to people who haven't tried it. This has been a very stressful year in general, with the events of September 11 in the city, and my mom's passing. Power-*of*-10 has been like an anchor in my life, keeping me in a very positive place.

Dr. Steven Kafko age 53

DENTIST

This Dentist Needed Novocain Just to Exercise—Then He Found Power-of-10 . . .

Over the last several years, I don't think my daily weight-training routine was producing anything you'd call progress. I would train and hurt my shoulder, train and hurt my knee. Just as I was making progress I would hurt myself again. I'm 5 feet 11 inches and 160 pounds. When I hit 50, I bench-pressed 200 pounds, which was a big deal to me. But then I was out of the gym for 4 to 5 months with a rotator cuff injury!

Dentists are prone to cervical spine problems. At one point, I had surgery and had a piece of my hip placed in there, and had a disk fused (diskectomy). The doctors were always telling me not to do dentistry, not to run, not to lift weights, not to work out, etc. Basically swim or do the stationary bike.

A few years later, Adam happened to open his gym a few doors from my office. So one day I decided to go over and see what it was all about. When I met Adam, I was captivated by what he had to say—especially about the inherent safety of his method. I really enjoyed the first workout. Once you start, you're not merely working your body, you're working your psyche, your brain. You have to concentrate and do things like remembering to breathe throughout the exercise. After a workout, it takes me a good hour to come down. It's like a runner's high. You start to really look forward to going that one day a week.

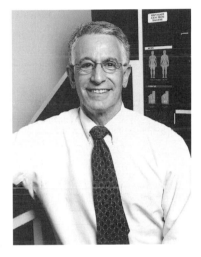

I've made tremendous improvement from a clinical perspective. I've increased my strength, but Power-*of*-10 has also helped me relieve stress and increase my focus, which was really important. Now I'm going once a week. I'm also doing fewer exercises, only 5 instead of 6 to 7. I keep getting stronger and gaining more lean muscle mass. I weigh about the same as I did before I started, but the difference is that my percentage of body fat went down from 18 to 10 percent. I've also stopped running. This is a big turnaround for me, as I used to run 25 to 30 miles per week. But my knees feel so much better, and I don't seem to have lost anything. In over a year with Power-*of*-10, I have no pain, I haven't missed a week, I've never hurt myself. I've never had disk problems, never looked back. When I go back to my doctors, they're really amazed.

Ron Storch age 35

CPA

A Distance Runner with "Runner's Knee" . . . Until He Tried Power-of-10 . . .

Before I met Adam I was a serious runner who also had serious knee problems. I was diagnosed with runner's knee, something you get when the hamstrings develop more than the quads, pulling your kneecap out of normal alignment. I was training for races and strength training at the gym 3 to 4 days a week to try to alleviate my problem. But even with the quad and hamstring workouts at the gym, I still was running in unremitting pain. Not only that, my schedule was crazy. Three small kids, a busy CPA practice, running, training—and when tax season hit, I went nuts.

Adam came to my CPA practice as a client. Naturally, we started talking about his business. He explained that with Power-*of*-10, he could cut my workouts down to once a week, and even allow me to shorten my daily runs because of the

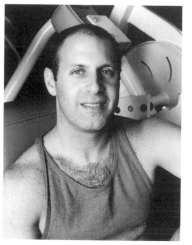

extra strength and endurance benefits. I was totally skeptical of course, but Adam didn't care if I believed him. He just said I had to find out for myself. So out of professional courtesy, I did.

The one thing I noticed immediately was the deep, complete feeling of the workout, like every fiber was being fired and nothing was being left on the table. I liked the idea that there was no explosion of force or swinging of weights in the movements, which can cause injury.

Within 4 to 6 weeks, something amazing happened. My knee pain actually began to fade until it just went away. All my previous work at the gym hadn't strengthened my quads the way Power-*of*-10 had—all from working out once a week. I was hooked.

Today my life is better in three ways. First, I'm getting all the exercise I need without a ridiculous time commitment at the gym. Second, I can run fewer miles and still get a full training effect because of the extra leg endurance I get from Power-*of*-10. In fact, I've started running marathons for the first time because I'm running faster and harder than ever before. And third, I have significantly more time for my family and other interests outside of pure training.

I'm 35 now and in the best shape of my life. I recommend Power-*of*-10 to anyone who will listen.

Please visit us at www.power-of-10.com (don't forget the hyphens) for the latest information on Power-*of*-10, including streaming video of your favorite exercises, nutrition, health tips, and much more.

INDEX